PRAISE FOR *CHILD HEALTH GUIDE*

"This book offers a fresh voice for parents and professionals in search of a wide-angle view of child health. Randy Neustaedter has given us a wealth of information collected from his extensive experience caring for children. *Child Health Guide* will be an invaluable addition to the field of Pediatrics for anyone who wishes to expand their knowledge beyond the confines of our conventional health care system."

—Stephen S. Cowan, M.D., FAAP, Pediatrician

"*Child Health Guide* provides parents and healthcare practitioners with valuable information to keep children healthy. This book teaches us to strengthen and maintain vitality in infants and children using natural interventions. Randy Neustaedter offers a strong voice to support another way of thinking about how we raise our children."

—Lawrence B. Palevsky, M.D., FAAP, Pediatrician

"Congratulations to Dr. Neustaedter on another great book! With sections on nutrition, sleep, behavior, common health problems, and more, *Child Health Guide* will prove an indispensable reference for parents wanting to raise their children in a more healthful, natural, and thoughtful way. While thoroughly researched and referenced, the concise presentation makes the information easy for busy parents to absorb and use right away. Dr. Neustaedter's dedication to the betterment of our children's health can be found on every page."

—Janet Lavatin, M.D., Pediatrician, and Clinical Instructor in Pediatrics at Harvard Medical School

"Well-researched, thought-provoking, practical, and an intelligent challenge to conventional medical views, Randall Neustaedter's book is a valuable resource for parents and pediatric professionals alike."

—Sabina Sonneman, M.D., Pediatrician

CHILD HEALTH GUIDE

RANDALL NEUSTAEDTER, OMD

HOLISTIC PEDIATRICS FOR PARENTS

North Atlantic Books
Berkeley, California

Published by
North Atlantic Books
P.O. Box 12327
Berkeley, California 94712

Cover and text design by Brad Greene
Printed in the United States of America
Distributed to the book trade
by Publishers Group West

Child Health Guide is sponsored by the Society for the Study of Native Arts and Sciences, a nonprofit educational corporation whose goals are to develop an educational and crosscultural perspective linking various scientific, social, and artistic fields; to nurture a holistic view of arts, sciences, humanities, and healing; and to publish and distribute literature on the relationship of mind, body, and nature.

Disclaimer: The following information is intended for general information purposes only. Individuals should always see their health care provider before administering any suggestions made in this book. Any application of the material set forth in the following pages is at the reader's discretion and is his or her sole responsibility.

North Atlantic Books' publications are available through most bookstores. For further information, call 800-337-2665 or visit our website at www.northatlanticbooks.com.

Substantial discounts on bulk quantities are available to corporations, professional associations, and other organizations. For details and discount information, contact our special sales department.

Library of Congress Cataloging-in-Publication Data
Neustaedter, Randall, 1949–
   Child health guide : holistic pediatrics for parents / By Randall Neustaedter.
     p. cm.
   Includes bibliographical references and index.
   Summary: "A complete medical resource book on holistic pediatrics and natural treatment for children"—Provided by publisher.
    ISBN 1-55643-564-9 (pbk.)
   1. Pediatrics—Popular works. 2. Holistic medicine—Popular works.
3. Children—Diseases—Alternative treatment—Popular works. I. Title.
RJ61.N387 2005
   618.92—dc22
                                                           2005004727

        2 3 4 5 6 7 8 9 UNITED 10 09 08 07 06

CONTENTS

Holistic Pediatrics, Defined

A practical approach to the philosophy of pediatric care that focuses on the principles of health, wellness, and the safe resolution of illness. Dedicated to integrating treatments that utilize natural methods to stimulate healing, recover balance, and support the body's own resilience.

—Holistic Pediatric Association

This book will tell you nearly everything you need to know about natural health care for your child. While many books discuss the holistic approach to parenting and raising children, no other book provides the necessary information parents need to make informed health decisions for their child, including choices about natural medical care. In this book I discuss the issues that affect your child's health just as I do with parents in my own practice. My approach to child health includes the philosophy of holistic pediatrics and the use of natural and alternative medicine. Holistic pediatrics promotes an inclusive understanding of physical, nutritional, environmental, mental, and emotional well-being as essential ingredients in maintaining the health of our children. The tools to create good health are well within your grasp, and my goal in this book is to provide you with the best guidelines for ensuring that your children are vibrant, healthy individuals.

Unfortunately, children today are exposed to innumerable toxic chemicals and drugs that deplete the system, lower resistance, and create lifelong illness. With the approach outlined in this book, you should feel confident that your child can have the best start to a lifetime of optimum health.

Health decisions fall into two categories: things to avoid because they are harmful, and things to do that will promote health and well-being. Most of these decisions involve common sense, once you have the necessary health information. My intention is to provide you with the concepts and data needed to make confident, informed choices. Above all, the safety of your child should be paramount, as the health choices you make today can have short- and long-term effects. We want to think about the future health of our children, so even when treating acute illness it is best to use methods that encourage healing and promote a stronger, more resilient system, rather than using drugs that suppress and weaken the body's defenses. In fact, acute illness provides an excellent opportunity to bolster the body's immune system.

For many issues I will provide recommendations and advice on nutrition, safeguarding your child's health, avoidance of toxins and specific drugs, and treatment for a variety of health problems. For other issues I will offer alternatives so that you can make your own choices based on balanced information. A parent's intuition and wisdom should always determine health decisions. I provide guidance and perspective to help you sift through facts and opinions, so you can arrive at your own determination of the best course to follow for your family.

Part I covers the basics. First, we'll look at the choice between conventional and natural health care, and how they can be integrated. Then we'll move on to nutrition—the most important foods and supplements for a lifetime of good health, as well as the foods and additives to avoid. Part I also covers daily decisions a parent makes that will affect a child's present and future health, including the chemicals and drugs that may undermine a child's resistance and constitution.

Part II takes you on a tour from birth through early childhood, reviewing healthy choices you can make along the way. You will find specific nutritional guidelines for different ages that are appropriate for each stage of child development. Part III describes simple and effective natural treatments for a wide range of childhood ailments that you as a parent can manage at home.

I wish you good fortune and fortitude in the rewarding, exceptional, and sometimes trying journey of parenthood. Above all, I wish you happiness with your children. I hope the information in this book will set you and your children on a path of good health and confidence in your medical decisions. I will provide you with many resources to guide you in areas of parenting and lifestyle choices, and I encourage you to read a wide range of books about children and child-raising, development, and emotional health. Knowledge will always help overcome anxieties in this daunting task of parenting. Seek other like-minded parents. Search for your own community of people who will support your decisions. With knowledge and a support network, you will find yourself fortified for the arduous and incredible journey ahead. I would like to be your partner in this adventure, and I will suggest many other partners to help you along the way.

—Randall Neustaedter

PART ONE

NATURAL CHILD CARE

CHAPTER I

The Basics

The Choice to Pursue a Natural Approach

Many parents are understandably dissatisfied with conventional pediatric care. Today's parents are concerned about their child's exposure to toxic chemicals, environmental hazards, and unnecessary medications. They question the accepted beliefs of previous generations concerning nutrition, extended breastfeeding, mandatory vaccination, bedsharing, educational expectations, and child discipline. This book provides parents with the tools to sort through the range of choices available to them and come to their own decisions about raising healthy children. The perspective of the *Child Health Guide* is always to promote health through natural means, to work with a child's natural defenses and his or her individual style of learning and behavior. Holistic parenting creates children with self-confidence and a foundation of emotional security. Holistic health care seeks to understand the underlying cause of illness while relieving symptoms with the safest and gentlest of treatments. A holistic pediatric approach will strengthen the body, repair imbalance, and build a resilient and efficient immune system.

The decision to pursue a natural or holistic approach may not be easy for parents. It may involve rejecting advice from grandparents, friends, and the pediatrician. It may be a struggle, but the rewards for your child are lifelong. The goal of holistic pediatric medicine is harmony and optimum health in children and families. Some decisions amount to simple, common-sense choices such as buying organic baby food, avoiding chemical additives, or choosing natural-fiber clothing. The decision to pursue a natural approach for children does not signify a rejection of everything that conventional medicine has to offer. Although rare situations may require the relatively high-tech methods of modern pediatrics, most childhood ailments can be managed at home with the simple, natural treatments described in this book. More serious acute illness may require the assistance of a qualified holistic practitioner. For a child whose chronic conditions such as asthma or diabetes necessitate the prescription of pharmaceutical medications, a holistic practitioner can develop a plan to also integrate natural therapies that encourage healing.

Parents have the ability, with a little diligence and understanding, to ensure optimum health for their children. A few simple choices can mean the difference between a child beset with allergies and recurrent ear infections and a child with a vital and resilient immune system. Prevention, cure, and optimum health are often elusive concepts in the conventional medical setting, but parents equipped with information about natural approaches have the advantage of making informed and educated decisions that can have permanent beneficial effects.

Integrating Conventional and Natural Treatment
A Parent's Role in Health Care Decisions

You want quality health care for your child—the best that modern medicine has to offer, when it's needed, and the most natural and nontoxic care available. It is your job to create an integrated medical team for your child's health care. This requires that you take an active role as medical manager and advocate for your child. In most situations, parents will see a pediatrician for well-child visits and serious medical problems,

---

NATURAL HEALTH CARE SYSTEMS

Homeopathic medicine A philosophy and form of medical treatment that uses natural remedies prepared from a plant, mineral, or animal substance capable of stimulating a healing response in the body. The medicines are prepared by pharmacies under FDA supervision. Practitioners should hold a CCH, DHANP, DHT, or RSHom certification in classical homeopathy.

Naturopathic medicine A form of natural medicine that includes training in holistic philosophy, nutrition, homeopathy, herbs, and Chinese medicine. Practitioners are graduates of four-year naturopathic medical schools and hold an ND degree, and should be licensed by your state's Naturopathic Medical Board.

Oriental medicine The use of herbs, acupuncture, acupressure, and oriental massage to create energetic balance in the body, practiced in accordance with principles developed in China and Tibet. Practitioners hold an LAc and/or OMD degree and should be licensed by your state's Acupuncture Board.

Chiropractic and osteopathic manipulation Two systems of body work that rely on manipulation of the spine and soft tissue to create balance in the body. Many practitioners also prescribe nutritional supplements and other forms of natural treatment.

---

but also practice home prescribing themselves for simple health problems. Many families will also consult a practitioner of natural medicine. More and more parents are also finding pediatricians and other primary care providers who have a holistic approach to pediatrics.

Natural treatment falls into one of several categories. First are home interventions such as herbs or over-the-counter homeopathic medicines for acute illnesses (colds, earaches, and chicken pox). The second type of natural treatment involves consulting a practitioner of homeopathy, naturopathic medicine, oriental medicine, herbalism, osteopathy, or chiropractic medicine for advice about illness or chronic problems. The third category includes maintaining a natural lifestyle that will promote health and prevent disease. The advantages of using natural methods include creating a strong immune system in your child, avoiding the adverse effects of drugs, and maintaining an optimal level of health. Taking a holistic approach to your child's medical care that includes promoting wellness, avoiding toxins, and using natural medical care to treat symptoms will establish a lifetime of health and balance.

You, as parents, are ultimately responsible for your child's health care decisions, and your medical providers offer advice and guidance. It helps if your providers are knowledgeable in holistic medicine, but if you cannot find a pediatrician amenable to alternative care, you can still pursue natural forms of treatment for your child's illnesses and symptoms. It is vital to remember that your pediatrician works for you. If you encounter a hostile or dismissive attitude from your doctor toward alternative medicine, do not be intimidated. You can still pursue the combination of care that you believe is the most beneficial for your child. Of course, in emergencies or times of critical illness you will need to trust in the advice and prompt treatment rendered by medical staff. Once your child's condition is stabilized, then you can supplement his or her care with natural interventions.

Knowledge is empowering. The more you know about your child's symptoms and the alternatives available, the more assured you will feel in your decisions. Keep good reference books at home and utilize the Internet to research specific concerns. Your natural anxiety about your child's symptoms will decrease as you develop an understanding of the problem. Then you can make decisions based on information. Consult with experts, gather your facts, and then choose the best course of action. Look at both sides of an issue, and decide for yourself the least toxic and most effective solution. Choosing an alternative to conventional pediatric care may involve rejecting the generally accepted mode of treatment. It takes courage to pursue an individual path, but your children will benefit from your convictions and your informed decisions about their health care.

The Role of Conventional Medical Care

Babies need medical checkups, approximately every three months in the first year, then less frequently as they grow, and once a year after age 2. A health care provider with an understanding of child development and pediatric medical problems needs to perform these checkups. This may be a pediatrician, family practice doctor, naturopathic physician, or other appropriately trained medical professional. The reason for these checkups is that problems may become evident that were not present or obvious at a baby's birth. Vision and hearing need to be checked, and blood tests for anemia and lead are often appropriate. Medical providers sometimes discover excessive wax or fluid in children's ears, hip or back problems, and genital abnormalities, none of which may be obvious to even the most attentive of parents.

Even when your pediatrician discovers a medical problem, you can still investigate alternatives to conventional treatment. If you have found a doctor who respects your desire to pursue the most natural and gentle forms of treatment possible, then communication can be open. You can utilize your pediatrician for information. Does my child have pneumonia? Are her eardrums red? Then you can decide what to do. Thank you, we will take the prescription for antibiotics and use them if it becomes necessary, but we'd rather try a more natural approach first. Some health problems—a broken bone, a severe asthma attack—require immediate conventional care, but with most symptoms you can take a watchful, waiting attitude while you pursue natural methods of care that do not involve a risk of side effects. Part III of this book delineates

---

QUESTIONS FOR THE PEDIATRICIAN

Do you feel comfortable with my using natural forms of treatment for my child's illnesses?

Would you support my using natural remedies for ear infections rather than antibiotics?

If I choose not to use some vaccines for my child, would this be a problem for you?

Do you support co-sleeping and extended breastfeeding?

---

those times when you should seek professional care so that you can feel confident about managing your child's symptoms at home.

Conventional medical treatment is often successful at relieving symptoms with drugs, managing life-threatening emergencies, and patching up essentially physical problems (with casts and stitches). However, conventional drugs have side effects and sometimes toxic effects that can interfere with the body's natural healing processes. If parents also utilize natural healing systems they will discover methods that heal the causes of medical problems and treat illnesses safely and effectively without side effects.

The Role of Natural Medical Treatment

If you have access to a practitioner of holistic medicine, first make sure that he or she is familiar with children's health problems and is knowledgeable in using natural therapies. Some practitioners do not treat infants and young children. The purpose of natural treatment is to strengthen the immune system and work with the body to overcome symptoms. Natural treatments may include homeopathy, herbs, acupuncture, and physical manipulation. These methods have no side effects because each system works by stimulating a healing response in the body, relying on the body's own healing mechanisms to overcome illness. The goals are permanent cure of chronic illness, nontoxic treatment of symptoms, and prevention.

The most problematic issue involved in the treatment of children with natural methods is remaining confident that serious symptoms are not being neglected. If your holistic medical provider is trained in diagnosis, then you will feel more confident. If you must handle natural treatment on your own with the help of books, then you will need to work with your pediatrician to remain within a margin of safety. In an obvious scenario, if your child has the cold that is going the round of your family, then treating her with homeopathic medicines, herbs, and nutritional supplements should not raise your anxiety level. However, if you suspect an ear infection, or if your child has a bad cough, then obtaining a diagnosis is essential. Part III of this book, on home treatment, will help you to decide when professional care is needed.

With a chronic illness you may need to balance natural treatment with conventional methods. Managing the interactions of natural treatment, such as homeopathy, with any kind of drug regimen requires skilled professional care. The most common reasons to consult a holistic practitioner are allergies, asthma, eczema, recurrent respiratory or ear infections, and behavior or attention problems. Homeopathy has earned an excellent reputation in the treatment of these conditions. A homeopathic practitioner will most likely schedule a one-hour evaluation visit and then prescribe a constitutional homeopathic medicine. The prescription may be a single dose of a high potency or a daily dose of a lower, or LM, potency. The homeopath will want to see the child again in two to four weeks for a follow-up visit. Constitutional prescribing requires experience and an understanding of homeopathic theory and case management principles. This is not the realm for parental home prescribing. Other interventions, including herbs, nutritional supple-

---

QUESTIONS FOR THE HOLISTIC PROVIDER

Do you have experience treating children?

Are you comfortable treating newborns and infants?

Do you have relationships with pediatricians who are supportive of your practice?

How do you handle emergencies? Are you available by phone when the office is closed?

---

ments, or acupuncture, may all be appropriate depending on the judgment and specialty of the practitioner.

Natural Treatment at Home

Appropriate home remedies for symptoms include homeopathy, herbs, acupressure, and nutritional supplements. Parents can learn how to use these treatments through this and other books or classes. No prior experience is necessary. These forms of natural treatment allow parents to take control of their children's health care, and provide parents with the assurance that mild symptoms can be alleviated without risking the side effects of drugs.

Homeopathy provides an especially effective and convenient way for parents to treat children's illnesses. Homeopathic medicines are completely safe and nontoxic, they work well when prescribed correctly, kids loves their taste so parents get no argument about taking a dose, and the remedies themselves have minimal cost. Homeopathy treats a wide range of acute problems including earaches, coughs and colds, fever, stomach flu, teething, hives, sprains, and many others. Homeopathic treatment will stimulate a healing reaction, encouraging the body to fight off an infection and correct an imbalance that causes symptoms.

Herbs can be more problematic for small children. Their taste is not

---

PREPARE A MEDICAL PLAN

Find a pediatrician or other provider to do well-baby checkups.

Find a holistic provider who uses natural treatments for times of illness and advises about prevention.

Purchase books on natural treatment for home reference.

---

always conducive to a cooperative attitude. Several Chinese herbal formulas have been developed specifically for children to relieve the symptoms of colds and congestion, coughs, digestive problems, and many other ailments. Western herbs have a wide range of uses, from coughs to parasites. Acupressure or Chinese meridian massage are also soothing techniques for specific symptoms such as colic or fevers. All of these methods are discussed in detail in Part III of this book.

Cornerstones of Healthy Child Care

The principles of raising children with a holistic pediatric approach are simple. The application of these principles can become complex. The remaining chapters of this book are dedicated to providing you with the tools to apply these principles.

Attachment parenting practices are based on the assumption and philosophy that a close relationship between you and your baby will result in a secure and confident child. *Close* means that you keep your baby close to your body nearly all the time. Attachment parenting implies three principles concerning the way you attend to your baby: breastfeeding on demand, babywearing, and bedsharing. None of these practices are new; people all over the world have applied these three principles

---

PRINCIPLES OF HOLISTIC PEDIATRICS FOR PARENTS

Apply the concepts of attachment parenting.

Feed your children natural foods.

Avoid toxins in your child's environment, skin products, and foods.

Treat illness and symptoms with holistic medical approaches.

---

to infant care since time immemorial. Breastfeeding on demand is an infant-centered response to your baby's natural needs. No external expectations or artificial schedules need to be engrafted on your baby's instinctual desire to nurse when hungry or for comfort. Babywearing means that you usually carry your baby with you in your arms, or in a sling or front carrier. This practice is taken for granted as appropriate in most cultures. Wearing babies in a papoose or a sling is the accepted and expected mode of mothering in most areas of the world. Keeping your infant close to your body at night during sleep helps ensure the baby's safety and health (see page 58.). Attachment parenting is primitive, natural, and sensible. Our culture has encouraged the separation of mother and baby for a number of reasons. We have mistakenly assumed that formula feeding is better than breastfeeding, discouraging mothers from sharing and exposing their breasts. We have isolated and neglected infants in separate rooms called nurseries. And we have incorrectly encouraged independence at an age when babies are completely dependent. None of these modern practices with infants help to develop healthy children. Babies need lots of touching, holding, and constant attention. Caring for your baby in this way is actually easier and simpler than instituting schedules and inflicting unnatural habits on this completely dependent and vulnerable little being.

Feeding your baby natural foods sounds sensible and straightforward. Why would anyone want to feed babies unnatural foods? Yet we do it all the time. Pesticides, preservatives, hormones, and drugs are often hidden in fruits, vegetables, and animal products. An infant's liver is simply unable to manage these toxins. Even older children have much less ability than adults to handle these toxic ingredients in our foods. If you feed your baby organic foods whenever possible, and feed your older children as few of these toxins in foods as possible, then you will be establishing a basis for resilience, fortitude, and strength, in both the physical and mental realms. Similarly, avoiding environmental toxins and harsh chemicals is only sensible. However, our homes, our bathroom cabinets, and our bathtubs contain products that can compromise a baby's health when she breathes or touches these chemicals. The following chapters provide all the information you will need to make your child's diet and environment as friendly and nurturing as possible.

When symptoms or illnesses occur in your children, you can treat most of them with methods that encourage healing, and use medical interventions that are gentle and life-promoting. It is best to avoid chemicals that suppress the body's own healing mechanisms unless they are absolutely necessary. A holistic approach to illness addresses the underlying imbalance in recurrent problems, and with it you will create a state of harmony, clarity, and excellent health in your child. Part III of this book will guide you to the best natural treatments for relieving acute illnesses with ease and safety firmly in mind.

Developing with Your Baby (a Note on Parenting)

A baby's different developmental stages will require different styles of parenting from you. The completely dependent 4-month-old needs more carrying and nursing than the roaming 9-month-old who feeds herself with a spoon. These stages obviously call for different kinds of parenting responses from you. You do not need a guidebook to tell you that. But parents are constantly falling behind their children. It is hard to keep up. Just when you become accustomed to one mode of behavior, priding yourself in your problem-solving skills, your child has already moved on to the next stage. Parents hear "don't treat me like a baby" all too often because they can't keep up with the dramatic changes that occur. Parents are constantly amazed at what their babies are able to do. Every day brings miraculous changes and new abilities. But all parents are conservatives and all children are revolutionaries. We want to conserve and preserve the moment, while they are aching to take the next giant leap ahead. Maintaining your equilibrium can be a daunting task.

I encourage you to read books about child development simply so you can be prepared for the next step. When your baby is pulling herself up to stand, read about toddlers. When your 10-year-old wants to ride his bike to the mall, read about teenagers. At least you will know what's in store. Be prepared with lists of job responsibilities appropriate for different ages and anticipate the appropriate freedoms to bestow upon your children depending on their maturity. Parents are guides, not adversaries. Don't get stuck in the role of bad cop. Use the tools of successful parenting. Have regular family meetings, discuss problems and solutions at times of low tension rather than during emotional storms, and use discipline wisely. Never hit your child. Children require nurturing, love, support, and respect, even in the most trying of circumstances. Do not betray their trust with punishments. You will only be met with fear and resentment, not the respect you seek and cherish.

Your growing child embodies a panorama of emotions, an ever-changing intellectual diversity, and a profoundly unique personality. Encourage your child's curiosity. Allow him to test limits. Stay one step

ahead and out of his way. Try to avoid power struggles. Provide guidance, but make allowance for mistakes. Maintain your sense of humor,
and enjoy your child now. Soon this amazing stage will pass and he
too will be grown.

CHAPTER 2

Nutrition Principles

Food Guidelines

Nutrition is a cornerstone of disease prevention and maintenance of good health in children. This chapter presents clear guidelines for parents to follow in choosing the right foods and avoiding foods that lead to disease and obesity. The nutrition principles discussed in this chapter are straightforward: Choose the most nutritious foods you can. Avoid toxic exposure and highly sweetened foods. Maintain a variety of foods in your child's diet.

Children may thwart these well-designed principles. They will gravitate to the sweetest foods possible. Our culture seems bent on subverting your best intentions, bombarding children with advertisements for sugary products that masquerade as a wholesome breakfast, and tempting them with candy tie-ins to their favorite cartoon characters.

Babies under age 1 have special nutritional needs. Specifically, they require fats as 50 percent of their diet, and they have a very difficult time digesting grains. The foods that children get in the first year will establish patterns of health for the rest of their lives. After age 1, nutritional requirements gradually change. An older child needs a much different diet than she did as a baby. Read Chapters 7 and 8 for the guidelines related to younger children. Most of the information in this chapter applies to children over 2.

Here are some suggestions for rules of the house.

- Do not keep candy in the house. If it is not there, children will eat it only on very unusual occasions. Your children may never develop a taste for sugar and chocolate if their exposure in early childhood is minimal.

- Buy packaged foods carefully, and read ingredient lists. Avoid foods with added sugar, corn syrup, and partially hydrogenated fats.

- Bake your own cookies, cakes, and pies. Use fruit as dessert.

You will find age-specific advice for feeding your children in Part II of this book. Here are some general suggestions for older kids.

- Offer your children a variety of healthy, nutritious foods.

- Keep fresh fruit readily available at all times.

- Provide choices at mealtime and do not be deterred by petulant refusals. Continue to offer foods even if your child has refused them in the past. Children will often become accustomed to a new food or taste only after repeated exposure.

Controversies abound in the area of children's nutrition. You will find conflicting advice in various books on child nutrition. The advice provided here is based on scientific understanding as we know it. Many rules for nutrition in other sources have been formed on the basis of accepted beliefs and cultural expectations. Unfortunately, the culture is a modern, Western model that includes fast foods, inordinate amounts of sugar, indiscriminate use of pesticides, and excessive carbohydrate consumption.

Be a nutritional role model for your children. If you eat well, basing your diet on healthy principles rather than cravings and addictions, then so will your children. There is rampant confusion about the role of carbohydrates in modern diets. While the USDA continues to promote low-fat, high-carbohydrate diets, a revolution of low-carb dieting and low-carb lifestyles is sweeping the Western world. The short-term results are nearly miraculous. The long-term results remain to be seen, but proponents of the low-carb revolution insist that this style of eating will return us to an era with limited heart disease and cancer deaths. Whatever the future holds in store for these predictions, one thing is clear: Adults need to decrease the amount of carbohydrates they eat as they age. What children need is a different question. Children clearly require a diet with a large percentage of calories coming from fats. Children also need the energy, fiber, vitamins, and minerals derived from whole grains. Most children need more carbohydrates in their diets than adults, although some children clearly do not respond well to gluten products and thrive on gluten-free diets.

Proteins in grain, especially gluten, are difficult to digest. Soaking grains will partially break down gluten and other proteins into simpler components that children can absorb more safely. Soaking grains also allows enzymes and helpful bacteria to neutralize phytic acid. All grains contain phytic acid bound to phosphorus in the outer layer, or bran. Untreated phytic acid combines with minerals including calcium and magnesium, blocking their absorption. For a more thorough discussion of cooking with grains, see *Nourishing Traditions* by Sally Fallon.

Children also need the vitamins and antioxidants they derive from fruits and vegetables. And, of course, children need protein and calcium. The remainder of this chapter will examine the important aspects of children's diets, what they should eat, and what they should avoid.

The food group portions guidelines for feeding children are based on the Rule of 3. This means three daily portions from the groups vegetables, whole grains, dairy, and animal products, plus three to six fruit portions each day, and some nuts or beans.

Food Group Portions, Applying the Rule of 3

Fruits:	3–6 per day
Vegetables:	3 per day
Whole grains (bread, pasta, cereal):	2–3 per day
Dairy (milk, yogurt, cheese):	2–3 per day
Animal products (chicken, turkey, beef, eggs):	2–3 per day
Nuts and beans:	1–2 per day

Serving sizes will vary depending on the size and age of the child. For a preschooler, a serving may be 1 or 2 slices of apple and 1/4 cup of yogurt. For an older child of 5 to 9, protein servings are 1 egg, 2–3 ounces meat, 1/2 cup milk, 1/2 ounce cheese, 1 tablespoon peanut butter, 1/4 cup beans; carbohydrates are 1/4 cup vegetables, 1/2 apple, 1 slice of bread, 1/4 cup pasta. Teens and adults can double these quantities as a serving. Some children have bigger appetites than others, a faster or slower metabolism, and different preferences. The important aspect of eating natural foods is to avoid overdoing any one food group and to keep the proportions more or less consistent.

Children with special dietary requirements will need to vary this list appropriately. Many children have food allergies and food sensitivities that necessitate elimination of individual or entire categories of foods. Some of these special needs will be addressed in the following pages. Others will require the advice of a trained and knowledgeable holistic pediatric health provider.

THE MOST IMPORTANT FOODS TO AVOID

Corn syrup and high-fructose corn syrup (stimulates overeating and interferes with mineral absorption)

Partially hydrogenated fats in cookies, crackers, and chips (promote allergies, inflammation, and heart disease)

Soy milk and soy products (deplete calcium and thyroid function)

Fish (mercury toxicity and PCBs in farm-raised and wild fish)

Artificial flavors, colors, MSG, soy protein isolates, and textured vegetable protein (excitotoxins and hormone busters that interfere with normal nervous system functions)

BASIC PRINCIPLES FOR HEALTHY EATING

Eat fresh fruits and vegetables, not bottled juices.

Use organic whole milk, yogurt, and butter when possible. The ideal milk to use is non-homogenized and raw/non-pasteurized.

Use chicken, turkey, beef, and pork raised without hormones and antibiotics.

Eat whole-grain breads and cookies, which contain more fiber and naturally occurring vitamins and minerals than those made with enriched wheat and bleached white flour. Organic wheat is best. Commercial wheat is heavily sprayed.

Avoid pesticides; feed your children organic, pesticide-free fruits and vegetables whenever possible.

Organic Foods and Pesticides

Pesticides pose several risks to children. They cause physical symptoms, impair mental function, disrupt hormone function, and increase the risk of developing cancer. Physical symptoms of pesticide exposure include respiratory problems and asthma, headaches, nausea, skin rashes, genetic damage linked to neurological disorders, and impaired immune function. Mental symptoms include disorientation, attention problems, and fatigue. Several types of cancers in children have been linked to pesticides, including leukemia, brain cancer, and soft tissue sarcoma.

Hormone disruption is an especially insidious effect of pesticides. Cells have hormone receptor sites that recognize specific hormones that will then trigger a response in the cell. Pesticides, and some other environmental chemicals like petrochemicals and plastics, can mimic hormones and bind to the same receptor sites, stimulating the same effects as hormones. Precocious puberty in young girls, for example, has been linked to pesticide and hormone exposure from foods. Fifty percent of African-American and 15 percent of Caucasian American girls now begin menstruating by age 8. All of this estrogenic activity also increases a woman's risk of developing breast and reproductive organ cancers. These same pesticides may also have the opposite effect, blocking hormones and causing infertility and masculinization of girls.

Pesticides from foods accumulate in children's bodies. A study published by the National Institutes of Health (NIH) has confirmed that children who eat a diet of predominantly organic foods have a much lower amount of pesticide exposure than children fed a conventional diet. The researchers measured by-products of organophosphorus pesticides in the urine of thirty-nine children fed organic and nonorganic diets. All children were aged 2 to 5 years old. Their parents kept a diet diary for three days and then provided twenty-four-hour urine samples for the study. The nonorganic group had six times the level of pesticide by-products compared to the organic group (Curl et al., 2003).

Children are much more likely than adults to develop toxic effects from pesticides. The Environmental Protection Agency (EPA) has drafted an assessment of cancer risk from toxic exposure in children. Based on animal studies and the dynamic action of carcinogens, the report estimates that children under 2 are ten times more likely to develop cancer from exposure to carcinogens than adults, and children between ages 2 and 15 are three times as likely (U.S. EPA, 2003). Small children have less ability to metabolize toxins, and children's exposure to environmental pesticides tends to be greater than adults' because of their increased exposure to floors, lawns, and playgrounds, more mouthing of objects, and because they breathe closer to the ground than adults. In addition, children have more skin surface for their size than adults to absorb environmental toxins.

The answer to this problem of pesticides is to limit children's exposure as much as possible. Never use commercial pesticides in your home or in your garden or lawn. Lobby in your community to stop the spraying of pesticides at schools. Finally, eat organic foods whenever possible.

Buy organic produce if you can. Clean commercially grown produce with a vegetable and fruit wash (available at health food stores, made from enzymes and surfactants that remove residual sprays on produce with skins). This is not a completely reliable method of eliminating pesticides because they may be absorbed into the body of the fruit or vegetable, but it helps.

Some fruits and vegetables have much more pesticide residues than others. A study from the United Kingdom showed that pesticide residues on some fruits are uncommonly high. Some apples, pears, raspberries, and grapes contained pesticides that exceeded the legal limits of permitted residues. The list goes on: Lettuce, cherries, and pumpkins also contained potentially dangerous levels of toxic pesticide residues. The produce originated from all over the world—grapes from Brazil and Europe, lettuce from Spain, and cherries from Canada (Pesticide Residues Committee, 2003).

The Environmental Working Group (EWG) has created a list of the

HIGHEST IN PESTICIDES

BUY ORGANIC OR UNSPRAYED:

Apples	Bell peppers
Celery	Cherries
Grapes (imported)	Nectarines
Peaches	Pears
Potatoes	Red raspberries
Spinach	Strawberries

LOWEST IN PESTICIDES

SAFE TO BUY FROM COMMERCIAL SOURCES:

Asparagus	Avocados
Bananas	Blueberries
Broccoli	Cauliflower
Citrus	Grapes (California)
Kiwi	Mangos
Melons	Onions
Papaya	Pineapples
Peas (sweet)	

A NATURAL FOODS DIET CURES TEENAGERS' BEHAVIOR PROBLEMS

Clinicians have been screaming about the effect of food on behavior and attention for the past thirty years. Long ago Feingold and Conners (of the Conners' Rating Scales) encouraged parents to delete the sugar, refined flour, and artificial chemicals from kids' diets. The value of this approach was dramatically demonstrated at a small school for problem teens in Appleton, Wisconsin. The Appleton Central Alternative High School was established in 1996 for troubled kids who could not attend traditional high school because of discipline problems. Things were so bad at Appleton Central that a police officer was stationed full-time at the school to prevent violence and weapons violations.

Then the owners of Natural Ovens Bakery donated $100,000 over five years to build a kitchen and hire a staff to provide a natural foods breakfast and lunch at the school, and everything changed. After the food program was initiated, the principal reported that students were calm, well-behaved, more receptive to learning, and happier. The school had no dropouts, no expulsions, no drug or weapons incidence, and no suicides in the three years since the program started.

What was the plan that achieved these drastic results? Soda, candy, chips, and chemically processed food items are absolutely prohibited in the school building. Meals provide an array of fresh produce, whole grains, and oven-baked entrees. Breakfast consists of an energy drink (made daily with fresh whole fruit, juices, and a flax-based powder), whole-grain breads and muffins (with no chemical preservatives), granola, fresh peanut butter, whole fresh fruit, and milk. For lunch students have access to a fresh salad bar with dark green lettuce and hot entrees that may include an oven-baked chicken patty with broccoli almandine rice, turkey in gravy with mashed potatoes and corn, or BBQ meatballs made from ground turkey with baked potato wedges.

Appleton, Wisconsin Healthy Foods Program: "Impact of Fresh, Healthy Foods on Learning and Behavior," 2002. A video about the program is available from Natural Ovens at www.naturalovens.com or by calling 800-558-3535.

most contaminated fruits and vegetables. The EWG recommends buying foods in the most contaminated group from organic sources. Other produce items are relatively safe from commercial sources with consistently low levels of pesticides. (For further information, check out www.foodnews.org.)

Whenever possible, buy animal products, including milk, eggs, chicken, turkey, beef, and pork, that are free of pesticides, antibiotics, and hormones. Organic eggs are readily available. Commercially raised chickens are housed in individual one-foot cages stacked in huge warehouses. They are fed a diet of antibiotics and grains laden with pesticides. Free-range chickens have access to the ground and to the outdoors. If they are labeled organic, then their feed contains no pesticides. Similarly, organic dairy cattle are fed no animal products and no pesticide-treated grass or grain. They are not treated with antibiotics. And they are given no growth hormones.

Beef and pork products should be free of hormones and antibiotics. Packaged meats should be nitrate and nitrite free. If you cannot get free-range poultry, then don't eat the skin. Pesticides tend to concentrate in the fat. The highest-quality beef is labeled organic. This means that the grain fed to the cattle in feedlots is free of pesticides.

Fats and Oils for Health

Children need fats. Low-fat foods can create fatty-acid deficiencies. Children especially need saturated fats and cholesterol to maintain healthy tissues and cell membranes. Cholesterol and saturated fats from breast milk, organic eggs, cream, coconut oil, and meats are essential parts of your child's diet. Children also need omega-3 fats for brain development. Breast milk contains the omega-3 fat DHA. Most children and adults eat too many polyunsaturated fats in the form of vegetable oils (omega-6 fats). Children get all the omega-6 essential oils they need from breast milk, grains, seeds, vegetables, and nuts. They should eat as little additional polyunsaturated oils in the form of vegetable oils as possible (corn oil, canola oil, safflower oil, etc.). A diet high in polyunsaturated oils impairs growth and learning, and promotes heart disease, cancer, and immune system dysfunction. The problem arises when polyunsaturated oils become oxidized after exposure to heat, oxygen, and moisture in processing and cooking. They release free radicals that attack cell membranes and damage DNA, initiating cellular and tissue damage that can promote tumor growth and inflammation of blood vessels with plaque formation (Fallon and Enig, 2001).

Saturated fats are necessary for calcium to be effectively incorporated into bones. At least 50 percent of dietary fat should be saturated (Watkins and Seifert, 1996). Omega-3 fats are retained better in tissues in the presence of saturated fats, and saturated fats promote healthy immune systems because of their antimicrobial properties that prevent the buildup of harmful microorganisms in the digestive tract. Contrary to accepted beliefs, saturated fats do not cause heart disease—they prevent heart disease and cancer.

Cholesterol acts as a precursor to vital hormones, including sex hormones and corticosteroids that protect the body against heart disease and cancer. Cholesterol is also a precursor of vitamin D that is essential to bone growth. Babies and children need cholesterol-rich foods to ensure proper development of the brain and nervous system (Fallon and Enig, 2001). Breast milk is especially rich in cholesterol.

Trans fats damage cell membranes, block the utilization of essential fatty acids, and promote disease (diabetes, heart disease, immune system dysfunction, and allergies). Trans fats must be artificially manufactured. Polyunsaturated fats are mixed with a metal (nickel oxide) and subjected to hydrogen in a high-pressure, high-temperature reactor. The hydrogen is forced to move in the fatty acid chain, creating an altered molecular structure. The normal *cis* structure of the oil is converted to its *trans* formation when the hydrogen atoms are forced to the opposite side of the chain. This straightens the chain, allowing the molecules to pack together more closely forming a solid that mimics saturated fats. The result is a partially hydrogenated oil, margarine, or shortening. Manufacturers of packaged foods love partially hydrogenated oil because it keeps products fresh and oily tasting, or keeps them crunchy or chewy. You will find it in most packages down the center aisles of the supermarket—in chips, crackers, cakes, croissants, and cookies. Beware of peanut butter with added partially hydrogenated oil as well. Trans fats will sit in cell membranes, creating a barrier that blocks the exchange of nutrients that promote health and chemicals necessary for efficient cell function. Trans fats prevent normal cell metabolism because cells can only function normally when the electrons in cell membranes are in certain arrangements or patterns. This arrangement is fatally altered by hydrogenation.

Fried foods are unhealthy because extreme heat damages fats. The damaged polyunsaturated oil and cholesterol release free radicals into the body that will in turn damage tissues and cells and promote disease processes. In addition, many fried foods are cooked with hydrogenated fats. Children should avoid commercial french fries, potato chips, and corn chips. These are not health-promoting foods.

Another problem with fried foods is the presence of a class of carcinogens called acrylamides. These are formed when starchy carbohydrates like potatoes, corn, oats, or wheat are subjected to high temperatures (above 360 degrees) for prolonged periods, as in deep-frying. Potato chips, doughnuts, and even oven-baked french fries contain acrylamide. This chemical is monitored in drinking water because of its ability to cause cancer.

By contrast, omega-3 fats have health-promoting and far-reaching preventive health effects. They create a flexible and permeable cell membrane that allows nutrients to pass easily into the cell. Omega-3 fats may be the key to prevention of heart disease, cancer, and arthritis, and the best thing going for allergies, asthma, and healthy brain functions.

Pregnant women and breastfeeding mothers should take a DHA-containing omega-3 supplement to ensure adequate levels of DHA (docosahexaenoic acid) in breast milk and adequate brain development in their babies. The DHA content of most American women's breast milk is lower than that in milk from women in other countries, and the DHA content of a woman's breast milk correlates with her dietary intake of DHA. Vegetarian women have the lowest levels of DHA in their breast milk (Fidler et al., 2000). When women supplement their diets with DHA in the form of fish oil, high-DHA eggs, or a DHA-containing algae capsule, the content of DHA in their breast milk increases. The increase in breast milk DHA also translates into higher DHA levels in infants (Jensen et al., 2000). In another study, infants whose mothers took fish oil supplements during pregnancy also had higher blood levels of DHA at birth than a control group that did not take a supplement (Connor et al., 1996).

It is difficult for children to get enough omega-3 fats from their diets once they are no longer breastfeeding. Children need to have supplements of omega-3 fats. The best sources of the omega-3 fats are cod liver oil (1 teaspoon per 50 pounds of body weight), fish oil capsules (containing 250 mg of DHA for children over 7 years old), and DHA supplements derived from algae (Neuromins). Chicken, eggs, and beef are also sources of omega-3 fats if the animals eat green plants and not just grains. Therefore, only cage-free chickens that eat green plants or algae and pasture-fed cattle are reliable sources. Small fish (anchovies, herring, and sardines) are another good source of omega-3 fats, but larger fish (tuna, shark, swordfish, mackerel, and salmon) may be contami-

DHA Supplementation

Pregnant/breastfeeding women	1 tablespoon cod liver oil per 150 lbs body weight
Infants	1/4 teaspoon cod liver oil per 12 lbs (5.5 kg) body weight
Children more than 3 years old	1 teaspoon cod liver oil per 50 lbs body weight, or 200 mg DHA from algae (Neuromins capsule), or 200 mg DHA from fish oil capsule

Cod Liver Oil Nutrient Content

In one teaspoon cod liver oil:

DHA	500–550 mg
EPA	460–550 mg
Vitamin A	1,000–1,250 IU
Vitamin D	400–500 IU

nated with mercury and harmful pesticides. Children should not eat these larger ocean fish or farmed fish (see page 48).

Flax seed oil is often recommended as an omega-3 supplement for children, but there is a problem. Flax seeds contain the omega-3 fatty acid ALA that must be converted to DHA by an enzyme so that the body can incorporate it into cells. Children make this enzyme only in small amounts, if at all. If they do not have the enzyme they will not benefit from the omega-3 fat in flax seeds. Newborns are completely unable to convert ALA to DHA. A study of breastfeeding mothers who took a flax seed oil supplement had no resulting increase in their own plasma or breast milk levels of DHA, showing that adults do not make this con-

FATS FOR CHILDREN

HEALTHY, IF FROM ORGANIC SOURCES: FATS TO AVOID:

Eggs   Partially hydrogenated oils (in chips,

Butter   cookies, crackers, cakes)

Coconut oil for cooking   Vegetable oils (polyunsaturated)

Whole dairy products   Fried foods
(in milk, yogurt, cheese)

Extra virgin olive oil for salads
and marinades

SOURCES OF FATTY ACIDS

OMEGA-6	OMEGA-3	OMEGA-9
Canola oil	Fish	Olives
Safflower oil	Algae	Avocados
Sunflower oil	Eggs (cage-free)	
Corn oil	Flax seeds	

FATTY ACIDS BY CATEGORY

OMEGA-6	OMEGA-3	OMEGA-9
LA (linoleic acid)	ALA (alpha-linolenic acid)	Oleic acid
GLA (gamma-linolenic acid)	EPA (eicosapentaenoic acid)	
AA (arachidonic acid)	DHA (docosahexaenoic acid)	

version either (Francois et al., 2003). Flax seeds are not an adequate source of DHA.

The only oils suitable for use at home are extra virgin olive oil (monounsaturated fat) for salads and marinades and coconut oil (saturated fat) for cooking. Olive oil will not cause any health problems, but it does not contain either of the two essential fatty acids LA or ALA. Coconut oil contains health-promoting lauric acid, which helps prevent infection and aids in the prevention of diabetes, heart disease, and cancer. Butter is also fine for cooking.

Vitamin E is a potent antioxidant that is also absorbed into cell membranes where it will prevent rancidity of fats that reside in the cell. In addition, vitamin E has anti-inflammatory effects and increases resistance to infection. Use only natural vitamin E (d-alpha-tocopherol), not the synthetic form (dl-alpha-tocopherol). A mixed tocopherol form of vitamin E is best. The dose for children 1 to 3 years old is 100 IU, for 4–12-year-olds 200 IU, and for teens 400 IU.

Omega-3 Fats Improve Attention, Behavior, and Intelligence

Several studies have demonstrated that children with lower levels of omega-3 fatty acids in their bloodstream have significantly more behavioral problems, temper tantrums, and learning, health, and sleep problems than do those children with high proportions of those fatty acids (Mitchell et al., 1987; Stevens et al., 1996). In a similar study, fifty-three children with ADHD had significantly lower proportions of key fatty acids (AA, EPA, and DHA) in their blood than did forty-three control subjects. Children with lower omega-3 levels had lower behavioral assessment scores (Conners' Rating Scales) and teacher scores of academic abilities (Stevens et al., 1995). The researchers speculated that an inefficient conversion of polyunsaturated fatty acids to AA and DHA may have been a significant factor in the lower levels of those fats in ADHD children.

In one study, researchers showed that children with ADHD were breastfed less often as infants than were the control children. They assume that the high levels of DHA in breast milk could be responsible for better performance later in life since infants are inefficient at converting polyunsaturated fats from other sources into the valuable omega-3 fat DHA that is essential for brain development. Even the duration of breastfeeding has been associated with higher intelligence and higher academic achievement in later childhood, and with higher levels of high school attainment (Horwood and Fergusson, 1998). A study published in 2002 also showed a significant association between intelligence levels in adults and the duration of their breastfeeding as infants (Mortensen et al., 2002).

The take-home message from these reports is to breastfeed your children and maintain adequate levels of DHA throughout childhood to encourage the best potential for successful academic performance and to reduce the possibility of learning and behavior problems.

Vitamin A

Retinol, or vitamin A, was first identified in 1907 by comparing rats fed protein and lard or olive oil for fat with rats fed a diet that added egg yolk or butterfat. The rats that ate the foods deficient in vitamin A failed to grow, but recovered with the supplemental foods. Only animal fats contain vitamin A. Good sources are cod liver oil, egg yolks, butter, raw whole milk, and liver. Animals must have carotene or vitamin A sources in their diets in order to produce vitamin A and pass it on to humans. There are no plant sources of vitamin A. Beta-carotene found in vegetables and fruits can be converted to vitamin A by the body in a ratio of 12:1. That is, it takes twelve units of beta-carotene to produce one unit of vitamin A. Infants and people with diabetes or poor thyroid function cannot make the conversion at all. Children convert beta-carotene to vitamin A very poorly. Therefore animal fat sources of vitamin A are essential for most of the population.

Vitamin A is needed for proper mucous membrane function. It is essential for the growth and repair of body tissues, and for efficient digestion of protein. Vitamin A promotes good eyesight, strong bones and teeth, and a vital immune system. White blood cells, T-lymphocytes, and every cell in the important mucosal barriers of the respiratory, digestive, and urinary tracts require vitamin A.

A diet containing significant amounts of fat will help ensure adequate vitamin A intake. Whole milk products, butter, and free-range eggs will help maintain necessary levels of this important nutrient. For those who may not be getting enough vitamin A, a supplement is essential.

The recommended daily amount (RDA) of vitamin A is 3,000 IU per day for adults (reduced from 5,000 IU) and 1,000–2,000 IU for children, depending on their age (1,000 at age 1, 2,000 by age 9). Primitive diets probably maintained ten times that amount. One egg contains 300 IU, one cup of whole milk or whole milk yogurt contains 225–250 IU of vitamin A. One tablespoon of butter contains 350 IU of A. The amount of vitamin A may vary by the season and the feed of the animals.

People eating a vegan diet are at a significant risk of vitamin A deficiency. It would take 6 cups of raw carrots or 20 cups of broccoli to obtain the recommended daily requirement of vitamin A per day.

Most everyone would benefit from a vitamin A supplement derived from fish oil. One tablespoon of cod liver oil contains at least 3,000 IU of A. Proper dosage is 1 teaspoon per 50 pounds of body weight. For adults with hypothyroidism or immune system problems (allergies, recurrent infections, autoimmune disease), a capsule supplement of 20,000 IU of vitamin A with vitamin D from fish oil may be appropriate.

The toxicity of vitamin A during pregnancy or at any other time applies primarily to synthetic (palmitate) rather than natural forms of vitamin A derived from fish oil (retinoic acid). Vitamin A in fish oil protects the body from toxicity. A study of people taking 300,000 IU of vitamin A per day for over a year revealed no adverse effects. However, the toxicity of vitamin A is very real, and children should not be taking excessive supplemental vitamin A.

There has been an association between vitamin A intake of 5,000 IU per day and an increased risk of osteoporosis. It is assumed that this increased risk is due to interference with the ability of vitamin D to maintain calcium balance. Taking vitamin D and other cofactors should mitigate this effect. Monitoring by a knowledgeable health care provider is important because of the complex interactions of nutrients including A, C, D, calcium, magnesium, and other minerals on bone health.

Vitamin D

When the American Academy of Pediatrics announced that all breast-fed babies should take a vitamin D supplement to prevent rickets, protests immediately arose from breastfeeding proponents who questioned the motives behind this denigration of breast milk's adequacy as a complete food for babies (Gartner et al., 2003). They also questioned the wisdom of universal supplementation for babies without adequate studies on possible adverse effects. Although vitamin D deficiency is most often associated with osteoporosis and poor bone development, many other health conditions have also been linked to low vitamin D levels. Two studies published in January 2004 showed that vitamin D intake significantly reduces the incidence of autoimmune disease. In one study, women who took 400 IU or more of vitamin D per day were 40 percent less likely to develop multiple sclerosis compared to women who used no D supplement (Munger et al., 2004). A second study showed a 33 percent reduction in rheumatoid arthritis incidence for women who took a vitamin D supplement (Merlino et al., 2004). Breast cancer, prostate cancer, skin cancer, depression, diabetes, and heart disease have all been associated with vitamin D deficiency. And, according to many authorities, vitamin D deficiency is all too common in North America and Europe.

Our bodies produce vitamin D in response to sunlight (UVB radiation), but areas of the world north of latitude 30 north—San Diego (USA) or Cairo (Egypt)—may not get enough sun during September through May to provide adequate vitamin D levels. The current recommendation for adult intake of vitamin D is 400 IU per day, but findings from a study published in the *Journal of Internal Medicine* suggested that a vitamin D intake of 600 IU was insufficient to maintain adequate vitamin D levels in the body in the absence of sun exposure. The researchers proposed an increase of the minimum daily recommended adult dose to 1,000 IU per day (Glerup et al., 2000). Others have suggested a healthy dose range of up to 4,000 IU of cholecalciferol, or D3 (Vieth et al., 2001).

Although vitamin D in extremely high doses can be toxic, studies have failed to find any toxicity from cholecalciferol (D3) in adults taking 4,000 IU, or even 10,000 IU, per day (Vieth et al., 2001). It is estimated that one full-body summer-sun exposure day will provide 50,000 IU of vitamin D. Despite these conclusions from research studies, the Food and Nutrition Board of the Institute of Medicine has set the tolerable upper intake level for vitamin D at 1,000 IU for infants up to 12 months of age and 2,000 IU for children, adults, pregnant, and lactating women (Institute of Medicine, 1999). Remember that vitamin D3 (cholecalciferol), the kind we get from the sun, has a much higher limit of safety than the synthetic form, vitamin D2 (ergocalciferol). This is because of the different biological mechanisms our bodies use to metabolize these two distinct chemicals, vitamin D2 and D3.

Babies

Babies' vitamin D stores at birth can be increased if their mothers have had adequate exposure to sunlight and/or adequate vitamin D intake during pregnancy. Vitamin D is essential for bone growth in infancy and throughout childhood. The two reliable and safe sources of vitamin D for babies are sunlight and cod liver oil. Although breast milk contains vitamin D, babies in Finland who are vitamin D deficient will not develop adequate levels of vitamin D from breast milk alone even when their breastfeeding mothers are supplemented with 1,000 IU of vitamin D (Ala-Houhala et al., 1986).

The World Health Organization has determined that a fully clothed infant without a hat would need two hours of sunlight a week, or about 17 minutes a day, to produce adequate vitamin D at 40° N latitude (Cincinnati or Beijing). An infant with only a diaper needs 30 minutes a week or about 4 minutes a day. Babies with medium to darker skin tones need a little more time in the sun (Butte et al., 2002). It is not necessary to get sun exposure every single day. The body will store vitamin D for extended periods of time (Good Mojab, 2002).

Avoid prolonged exposure to bright sunlight because of the danger of sunburn. Babies will get enough vitamin D if they have access to a bit of sun each day. Babies that reside in North America and Europe may need vitamin D supplementation during the colder months of the year when sun exposure is not possible and weather prevents adequate exposure to the healthy rays of the sun.

Cod liver oil will provide vitamin D, vitamin A, and the omega-3 fats that stimulate brain development. Give 1 teaspoon for each 50 pounds of weight. A baby that weighs 10 pounds should get 1/4 teaspoon, and a baby that weighs 20 pounds should get a little less than 1/2 teaspoon per day in the winter months. Use a source of cod liver oil that has been tested for contaminants and oxidation. Cod liver oil should not taste fishy; this is a sign of rancidity. In the late spring through early autumn, give 100 mg of the omega-3 fat DHA from algae (Neuromins) or a fish oil supplement without vitamin D to babies who are eating solids. Babies that are solely breastfed do not need additional DHA if their mothers have an adequate intake of omega-3 fats, such as a fish oil or cod liver oil supplement. Breast milk normally has high levels of DHA, which can be increased by taking an omega-3 supplement.

Do not use a daily sunscreen. Reserve sunscreen use for the prevention of sunburn during midday exposure in bright sunlight, when swimming, at the beach, and during snow sports. Then use only zinc oxide and titanium dioxide sunscreens either in a cream (Lavera, Dr. Hauschka) or micronized powder (ColoreScience).

To summarize babies' dosage of vitamin D: Sun exposure of 20 minutes per day fully clothed without a hat. When that is not possible, give 1 teaspoon of cod liver oil for each 50 pounds of weight. A baby that weighs 10 pounds should get 1/4 teaspoon, and a baby that weighs 20 pounds should get a little less than 1/2 teaspoon per day in the winter months. Do not give cod liver oil when adequate sun exposure is possible.

Milk and Calcium

Cow's milk has been promoted as a perfect food for children—high in protein, calcium, and healthy calories. On the other hand, milk's detractors, including knowledgeable physicians, have noted milk's many problems. Cow's milk ingestion has been associated with allergies, anemia, autism, diabetes, and cancer. What should parents do? Let's try to sort out the issues.

First, I do not recommend cow's milk until children are at least 18–24 months old (unless they still need a milk-based formula when weaning from breast milk). Breast milk is the best food for babies. Introduce yogurt first because its enzymes and bacteria result in a more digestible product. If no obvious symptoms occur, then try milk.

Dangers from Processing and Chemicals

Like most foods, the nutritional quality of milk suffers considerably during processing. Homogenized fat becomes inaccessible, and we need the fat in milk to absorb calcium. Pasteurizing milk kills bacteria essential for its digestion, converts lactose to an indigestible form, interferes with calcium absorption, and destroys vitamins A, C, and B complex.

For more information about raw milk, go to www.realmilk.com, where you will find nutritional information and sources of raw milk in your community (in the USA and around the world). Call your local health food store and ask about raw milk availability.

If possible, feed your children raw milk for adequate bone growth and the prevention of tooth decay.

Beware of low-fat or non-fat milk that contains added powdered milk solids. These are highly processed products, exposed to extreme heat, oxidized, and treated with a number of chemical additives known to be harmful to children. Non-fat dried milk, frequently added to low-fat milk, is high in nitrites, so avoid milk with added dried milk.

Avoid milk that contains bovine growth hormone, antibiotics, and pesticides. That means you should drink only organic milk. These chemicals may be responsible for some of the health problems associated with milk. Use organic dairy products (ice cream, cheese, yogurt) whenever possible.

And remember to avoid soy products (see page 51).

Protein

Milk is a concentrated protein food: 8 grams of protein in one cup of milk or yogurt, 6 grams of protein in one ounce of cheese. But a protein enzyme (xanthine oxidase) contained in milk has been associated with an increased risk of heart disease if the enzyme is absorbed intact into the bloodstream. This occurs when drinking homogenized milk because small fat globules surround the enzyme, preventing the body from breaking it down. Drink milk that has not been homogenized.

Milk protein molecules are large and irritating to the intestinal tract, which can result in microscopic intestinal bleeding and anemia. When milk protein molecules leak through the intestinal lining into the bloodstream they can initiate an allergic response. Symptoms of milk allergy can include chronic nasal and sinus congestion, asthma, and frequent ear infections with persisting middle ear fluid congestion.

Vitamin D Content

Butterfat contains a natural vitamin D complex. Vitamin D is needed for calcium absorption, and the body will produce vitamin D from sun exposure, therefore during winter months many people become deficient in vitamin D. A synthetic form of vitamin D is often added to milk (vitamin D_2, ergocalciferol), but vitamin D_2 is associated with liver toxicity. Those who live in areas with cloudy winter skies and cold weather should take natural vitamin D_3 (cholecalciferol), either in a supplement or in cod liver oil.

Calcium Content

A cup of milk or yogurt contains more than 200 mg of calcium. The problem is milk's high phosphorus-to-calcium ratio, which tends to cause calcium excretion. A solution to this problem is to supplement a child's diet with calcium citrate in the form of a liquid calcium-magnesium

Recommended Calcium Intake for Children

1–3 years old	500 mg per day
4–8 years old	800 mg per day
9–18 years old	1,200 mg per day

Calcium Sources (in mg per 100 grams or 3.5 oz)

Milk	120
Yogurt	120
Cheese	700–900
Tahini	600 (60 mg per 10-gm serving)
Broccoli	100
Spinach	95
Almonds	235 (or 23 mg in nine almonds)
Beans	50
Eggs	30 in each egg

supplement or chewable tablets. Fat is required to absorb minerals and vitamins in milk, so children should drink only whole milk and eat whole milk yogurt, not low-fat products. Vitamin C assists in calcium absorption, so eating fruits that contain vitamin C or taking a supplement will help.

Summary

If children are eating dairy products, use only organic whole milk and yogurt, preferably not homogenized. Buy raw milk if possible. Do not switch to low-fat milk products as children get older. Children need fat, and the cholesterol in milk is beneficial. Supplement children's diets with 500–1000 mg of calcium citrate, depending on age and other calcium sources. Give an omega-3 fat supplement to facilitate calcium absorption. Consider using a vitamin D supplement during the winter months.

With all of milk's problems, you may want to use alternatives. Do not use soy milk, however, because soy depletes the body's calcium and tends to decrease thyroid function. Almond milk is a good alternative because it contains protein and fat. Children with a family history of allergies, however, may develop allergic reactions to nuts, so rice milk would be a better choice. Rice milk is a less desirable alternative because it is almost solely carbohydrate and contains phytic acid, which also interferes with calcium absorption. Both almond and rice milk are low in calcium.

The best non-dairy sources of calcium are dark green vegetables and sesame seeds (tahini). Since children are unlikely to consume these foods on a regular basis, a chewable or liquid form of calcium citrate or calcium lactate is a good idea for all children. Interestingly, vegetarian populations with a low dietary calcium intake tend to have a higher bone density than their Western counterparts, but this may result from diets also being low in calcium-depleting substances (caffeine, refined sugar, red meat, and soft drinks).

If your child has problems with chronic congestion and/or ear infections, try stopping all dairy products for a month as you introduce other supplements and treatments to build immune function. Then if symptoms improve, try reintroducing milk products after a few months to evaluate their effect. Digestive problems (stomach aches and gas) may be caused by lactose (the sugar found in milk products) in children who are deficient in lactase (the enzyme that breaks down lactose). Taking lactase as a supplement when eating a meal with dairy products may prevent these symptoms.

Sugar and Sweeteners

Many books have been written about the dangers of sugar consumption and its ability to depress the immune system, impede cellular function, and stimulate the overgrowth of candida (yeast). Even the U.S. government is campaigning to reduce sugar consumption because of the alarming increase in American obesity. Sugar-buster and high-protein diet gurus have attained best-seller status insisting that sugars and other carbohydrates stimulate excess insulin production that results in storage of sugars in fat cells, wildly fluctuating blood sugar reactions, and an increased incidence of cancer, heart disease, and osteoporosis. Excess sugar consumption interferes with the body's absorption of minerals (calcium and magnesium), raises cholesterol levels, and causes allergies, kidney damage, high blood pressure, and a host of other problems. This knowledge has led to the concept of low-carbohydrate diets to control weight and prevent or cure disease. Nonetheless, children love sweet tastes, and children have a higher need for carbohydrates than adults. No one should eat added sugars on a regular basis. The sugars contained in fresh, natural foods are adequate to provide for everyone's energy needs. If you must have additional sweets in your diet, here is a review of your options.

Sugar Sweeteners

Refined sucrose (white sugar) made from plants (beets or cane) is depleted of vitamins and minerals during the refining process, which also adds several potentially toxic chemicals (bleaches and stabilizers). Natural sugars in the form of rice syrup, malt syrup, and raw honey are purported to have more nutritional value, but do nothing to reduce the deleterious effects of eating sugar.

High-fructose corn syrup is twenty times sweeter than sucrose, cheaper to make, and convenient for food manufacturers because it retains moisture and blends well with other ingredients. The free fructose in corn syrup interferes with the heart's use of minerals, depletes the ability of white blood cells to defend against infections, and raises cholesterol and triglyceride levels. Fructose inhibits the hormones that make us feel full (insulin and leptin), and it triggers the hormone that makes us feel hungry (ghrelin). Children do much better on diets free of corn syrup. Most commercial, sweet, processed food products contain high-fructose corn syrup. These products include candy, soda, energy bars, sweetened yogurt, energy drinks (Gatorade), and baked desserts.

Honey should be used only in its raw form because the heating process destroys enzymes and vitamins natural to the honey. Honey stimulates insulin production with the same mechanism as other forms of sugar. Do not give honey to infants under 12 months of age because of their inability to defend themselves against botulinum spores that may contaminate honey.

Maple syrup made from the sap of maple trees is up to 60 percent sucrose. It is essential that consumers use certified organic maple syrup because of the danger of chemical residues from forests sprayed with pesticides. Additionally, many maple syrup producers use formaldehyde pellets in the sap holes to prevent the holes from closing and formaldehyde in holding tanks as a preservative. Chemical anti-foaming agents may also be added to non-organic maple syrup.

Malt syrup is made from barley and contains primarily maltose, which is less than half as sweet as sucrose. **Rice syrup** is made from barley and rice. **Date sugar** is simply ground, dehydrated dates. Health food products often contain these natural sweeteners in packaged products.

Artificial Sweeteners

Artificial sweeteners seek to provide the sweet taste of sugar without raising blood glucose levels. These alternatives to sugar tend to be hundreds of times sweeter than sucrose. Their safety has always been a matter of controversy. Studies have both indicted **saccharin** (available as Sweet 'N Low) as a carcinogen and exonerated saccharin as safe. However, U.S. government reports of known carcinogens have continued to include saccharin in their lists since 1981. **Aspartame** (Nutrasweet, Equal) has been roundly condemned by many sources as a dangerous toxin capable of inducing hundreds of symptoms. It has been affectionately nicknamed Nutradeath. Besides causing headaches, allergic reactions, and symptoms that mimic autoimmune diseases, aspartame causes the accumulation of formaldehyde in the brain and other tissues, resulting in damage to the nervous system and immune system.

Because of the negative publicity about these sugar-free sweeteners, other alternatives have been developed. The newest kid on the block is sucralose (Splenda).

Sucralose is made by chlorinating sugar (sucrose). Three chlorine atoms substitute for three hydroxyl groups. Although Johnson & Johnson, the makers of Splenda, claim that sucralose is not absorbed by the body, the FDA has determined that up to 27 percent of ingested sucralose is absorbed. Other chlorinated molecules, such as the chlorinated pesticide DDT, are accumulated in body fat. Similarly, up to 30 percent of absorbed sucralose is metabolized and concentrated in the liver and kidney. Research in animals has shown that sucralose can result in shrunken thymus glands (up to 40 percent shrinkage), enlarged liver and kidneys, reduced growth rate, and decreased fetal body weight. No long-term or independent studies on sucralose have been conducted on humans, and no organizations are monitoring health effects. Many individuals have reported adverse effects of sucralose, including anxiety, panic attacks, headaches, pain (in nerves, joints, and chest), allergic type reactions, and diarrhea.

Xylitol is a five-carbon rather than a six-carbon sugar (glucose, fructose). It is referred to as a sugar alcohol. The body produces several grams of xylitol every day, and ingested xylitol is converted to glucose. Many bacteria cannot metabolize xylitol, and its presence is harmful to some bacteria. For that reason it is promoted in sugar-free chewing gum to prevent plaque buildup and cavities. It contains the same number of calories as sucrose, but is absorbed more slowly. Sugar alcohols do raise blood sugar levels, though not as much as sugar. Stomach cramping and diarrhea are potential side effects of xylitol and other sugar alcohols. Sugar alcohols draw water into the intestines. For this reason they can also promote dehydration and loss of electrolytes. Eating a large amount of sugar alcohol-sweetened food and then exercising could create problems with muscle cramping and heat stroke.

Sorbitol and **mannitol** contain six carbons, like fructose and glucose, but with an additional hydroxyl (alcohol) group that make them independent of insulin metabolism. Sorbitol, a natural ingredient contained in many fruits (prunes, apples, pears, peaches), can cause diarrhea. The Center for Science in the Public Interest (CSPI) has petitioned the FDA to require foods containing one or more grams per serving of sorbitol or other sugar alcohols, such as mannitol, to carry the following label: "NOTICE: This product contains sorbitol, which may cause diarrhea, bloating, and abdominal pain. Not suitable for consumption by children. To protect yourself, start by eating no more than one serving at a time."

Plant-Derived Sweeteners

Stevia is an herb native to South America and Asia. It has no calories and manufacturers claim that the plant actually has health benefits. It contains vitamins and minerals. It lowers high blood pressure, discourages bacterial growth, and improves digestion. Some people object to its mildly bitter taste, but others find it perfectly palatable. Some brands are more bitter than others. Try KAL brand stevia extracts (liquid or powder).

Stevia has not been approved by the FDA as a sweetener because animal studies showed fertility problems, including reduced sperm production, increased testicle growth, and small offspring in rats. In the laboratory, steviol can be converted into a mutagenic compound, which may promote cancer by causing mutations in the cells' genetic material (DNA). Researchers, however, do not know if this conversion occurs in humans.

Lo Han Kuo fruit extract (available as SlimSweet), made from a Chinese fruit-bearing plant, has zero calories and does not stimulate insulin reactions, but very little data exists about adverse effects. It is presumed to be safe, and is purported to be 200 times sweeter than sucrose. The conversion for recipes is 1 teaspoon of Lo Han for 1/2 cup sugar. Lo Han works very well in dairy recipes such as custard and hot chocolate, but not very well in baking.

Ki-sweet is made from kiwis and is purported to cause fewer insulin reactions than other sugars.

Conclusion

Many commentators on the sugar controversies have suggested a novel proposal: Avoid all sweeteners whenever possible. Rely on fruit for that sweet taste you (and your children) crave so you do not have to worry about depleting vitamins and minerals. Fruit contains natural antioxidants, which will also help to counteract the negative consequences of eating other sugars.

Children become easily accustomed to foods in their diets. Feeding kids sweet foods will lead to more sweet cravings. Children are especially susceptible to the adverse effects of chemical additives, so avoid the harmful artificial sweeteners in kids' diets. Try using Stevia or Lo

WHICH SWEETENERS ARE (RELATIVELY) SAFE?

Raw honey (Do not give any honey to infants under 12 months of age because they cannot defend themselves against the presence of botulinum spores)

Organic raw sugar (sucrose)

Organic maple syrup

Stevia

Lo Han (SlimSweet)

Xylitol, mannitol, maltitol

SWEETENERS TO AVOID

Refined sugar (sucrose)

Corn syrup and high-fructose corn syrup

Sucralose (Splenda)

Aspartame (Nutrasweet, Equal)

Saccharin (Sweet 'N Low)

Han extract to sweeten baked products for kids. Raw honey and organic maple syrup also make excellent toppings for that special treat.

Fish Unsafe for Children

Unfortunately, most fish is unsafe in any amounts for children. Salmon and other fish contain healthful omega-3 fats, but the amount of mercury and pesticides is so high in fish that it renders them unsafe as a food. When wild fish eat algae and other creatures that also eat algae, they will produce omega-3 fats. That's why Eskimos have such a low incidence of heart disease. But farmed fish are usually fed grains, so their omega-3 fat content is low. "Atlantic salmon" is a code name for fish raised on farms in Chile. Fish raised in this way are usually kept in over-crowded conditions and require antibiotics to keep them alive. Their meat will contain these antibiotics and any pesticides used to farm the grain.

Most salmon consumed in the U.S. (and other Western countries) comes from fish farms where the fish are fattened with ground fish meal. The Environmental Working Group (EWG) has discovered that the small fish used in the fish meal have absorbed PCBs (polychlorinated biphenyls) that are concentrated in the fat of farmed salmon. PCBs, used as industrial insulators, have been banned in the U.S. since 1976 because they cause cancer, impair brain development, and weaken immune function. But PCBs persist in the environment. Three independent studies have found PCB contamination in nearly every sample of fish meal tested. The EWG reports that farmed salmon contain concentrations of PCBs that are five to ten times higher than those found in salmon fished from the ocean. In addition to the 110 different PCBs, farmed salmon contains higher levels of 151 other chemical contaminants than wild salmon. Farmed salmon also contains higher levels of antibiotics, and the fat of farmed salmon contains 35 percent less omega-3 fats than wild salmon.

Wild fish, however, are not safe either because of their mercury content. Industrial wastes that contain mercury find their way into rivers, lakes, and oceans. Algae absorb the toxic metal as an organic compound. Then fish absorb the mercury when they eat the algae. Cumulative doses ingested from contaminated fish can result in mercury toxicity. Fish is therefore not safe for pregnant women either.

Researchers know that mercury compounds are toxic to babies as they grow in the womb, but there has been little evidence that older

children also suffer developmental problems after exposure to the poison. This could change after a study of the health of children on the
Faroe Islands in the North Atlantic, where inhabitants eat lots of seafood
and whale meat and so are exposed to relatively high levels of mercury.
The research group found that the children, when 7 years of age, had
a slower than normal transmission of electrical signals along a particular circuit in their brain and that this disruption became even worse
when the children were 14 years old after a continued diet of fish and
whale meat. The findings suggest that any harm done by mercury before
birth or in early childhood was not repaired as the children grew up.
And continued mercury exposure may continue to affect the brains of
teenagers (Murata et al., 2004).

I advise you to feed your families only wild Alaskan salmon and limit
your consumption even of that food source to once a month because
of the potential mercury content.

The good news is that several companies are producing "organic," or
cleaner, farmed salmon. The USDA does not have guidelines or certification for organic seafood, so technically the fish cannot be certified as
organic yet, even though some stores are using that term. The producers say that the fish are raised in a cleaner environment with more room
to swim, and are fed better food than those raised with conventional
farming practices, with no antibiotics or hormones. The producers do
not use chemicals to clean their nets. Some farms use a pigment to color
the salmon meat, and their feed may or may not be organic.

Two firms are primarily responsible for the newer, cleaner farmed
salmon. Creative Salmon Co. in British Columbia does not use organic
feed, but their fish meal is screened for PCBs and other contaminants.
They do use a synthetic carotenoid to color the salmon's flesh. Martin
International in Scotland uses organic fish meal and grain. No pigment
is added since their fish are naturally colored by marine creatures in the

feed. Neither company uses antibiotics, hormones, pesticides, or anti-fouling substances (Ness, 2004).

Soy Unsafe for Children

Soy beans and soy products are not appropriate foods for infants or children. Not tofu, soy milk, or soy formula. Not soy hot dogs, sausages, soyburgers, or textured vegetable protein. Not ever. Although soy has been promoted as a health food and an excellent alternative protein source with numerous health benefits, the proven adverse health effects of soy in children far outweigh any positive or philosophical reasons to eat soy products. Soy proponents claim that soy can lower cholesterol, prevent heart disease and breast cancer, and reduce bone loss in menopause. But farmers are cautioned not to feed growing domestic animals a diet high in soy protein. Pigs, whose digestive tracts are very similar to humans, are allowed only 1 percent of their feed as soy because of the risk of adverse effects on digestion and immune function (Bee, 2000). Soy product consumption has been linked to a long list of diseases and hormone dysfunctions in children, including thyroid disease, mineral malabsorption, diabetes, and abnormal sexual development.

Soy foods depress thyroid function. This depression of the thyroid gland is capable of inducing a hypothyroid state, autoimmune thyroid disease, and goiter (swelling of the thyroid gland). Soy beans contain compounds that inhibit thyroid peroxidase-catalyzed reactions that are essential for the production of thyroid hormone (Divi et al., 1997).

Soy formula feeding in infants is associated with thyroid disease. A review of children with autoimmune thyroid disease showed that these children had a higher frequency of soy formula feeding in infancy than their siblings or healthy control children (Fort et al., 1990).

Soy formula feeding is associated with hormone disruption. A study conducted in Puerto Rico of children with premature breast development found an association between the affected children under age 2 and soy-based formula as well as the consumption of meat products (Freni-Titulaer et al., 1986). Phytoestrogens (isoflavones) in soy products disrupt fertility (Irvine et al., 1995) and lower testosterone levels (Sharpe et al., 2002). Some researchers are concerned that soy formula given to infants can disrupt hormones at a crucial time for the programming of a baby's reproductive development. The testosterone surge in the first few months of life programs male infants for puberty and sexual development. If receptor sites intended for the hormone testosterone are occupied by soy estrogens, appropriate development may not take place (Santti et al., 1998; Winter et al., 1976).

Soy interferes with absorption of calcium, magnesium, zinc, and iron. Phytic acid blocks the uptake of essential minerals in the intestinal tract, and soy has one of the highest phytic acid levels of any grain or legume (Reddy and Sathe, 2002). Only fermentation of soy products in the preparation of miso, soy sauce, and tempeh removes the phytates responsible for mineral depletion.

Soy feeding in infancy has been linked to diabetes. When reviewing the feeding histories of ninety-five diabetic children, twice as many of the children with diabetes received soy formula in infancy compared to children in the control group (Fort et al., 1986). The American Academy of Pediatrics advised against the use of soy formula due to the diabetes risk (AAP, 1994).

Beware of soy additives in processed or packaged foods. Processed soy goes by several names, including textured soy protein, soy protein isolate (SPI), and soy isoflavones. These ingredients are added to many health food products and protein supplements. Soy is a primary ingredient of low-carb diet foods and protein bars. It is added to prepared frozen meals, ice cream, breads, and canned foods. Read ingredient list

---

WHY AVOID SOY?

Depresses thyroid function

Disrupts sex hormone functions

Blocks calcium and other mineral absorption

Linked to diabetes, breast cancer, and leukemia

---

labels and avoid soy-fortified foods and these protein substitutes for your children.

Nutritional Supplements

I do not recommend a routine multivitamin supplement for children. I do recommend some specific nutrients to supplement the diet if needed to maintain good health. Children who eat a healthy diet do not need supplementation with multivitamins, and the vitamin content of foods is far superior to the vitamins packed into supplements.

One study published in *Pediatrics* suggests that multivitamin supplementation may even be associated with an increased risk of babies developing asthma and food allergies. Infants given vitamins in their first six months showed a significantly higher incidence of food allergies if they were exclusively formula-fed, and 3-year-olds who used vitamins had an increased risk of food allergies whether they had been breastfed or exclusively formula-fed. Black infants had an increased risk for asthma if they took vitamins. Other known factors that increase the risk of asthma and food allergies were identified and taken into consideration (Milner et al., 2004).

Rely on fresh fruits, grains, beans, nuts, and whatever vegetables

DAILY DOSAGE OF SUPPLEMENTS FOR KIDS

	2–3-YEAR-OLDS	4–12-YEAR-OLDS
OMEGA-3 FATS:		
Cod liver oil	1/2 teaspoon per 25 lbs of body weight	
DHA (fish oil or Neuromins)	100 mg	200 mg
FAT-SOLUBLE VITAMINS:		
Vitamin E (d-alpha-tocopherol or mixed tocopherols	100 IU	200 IU
Vitamin A (from fish oil)	1,000 IU	2,000 IU
Vitamin D (from fish oil)	200 IU	200 IU
MINERALS:		
Calcium	250–500 mg	500–800 mg
Magnesium	250 mg	250–400 mg
Zinc	10 mg	20 mg
Copper	1 mg	2 mg

your child will eat. These should supply an adequate amount of water-soluble vitamins and antioxidants. Eggs, butter, milk, yogurt, cheese, and meats should provide vitamin A, cholesterol, saturated fat, calcium, and adequate protein. If your child refuses or cannot eat some of these food sources, you may want to add supplements to compensate. In the colder months and whenever sun exposure is inadequate, children should receive **vitamin D** (see page 35).

KIDSHAKE RECIPE

ADD THE FOLLOWING TO THE BLENDER, AND BLEND FOR A MINUTE OR SO:

3/4 cup organic rice or cow's milk (you can use organic cow's milk if your child is more than 2 years old)

Half a banana

1/2 cup frozen mango or other fruit (not strawberries unless organic—too many pesticides used on berries)

1/2 to 1 tablespoon liquid calcium-magnesium formula (equivalent to 300–600 mg calcium, if using rice milk)

1/2 teaspoon honey or maple syrup (optional, and use honey only if your child is more than 12 months old)

1/2 teaspoon vitamin C powder (optional, equivalent to 1,000 mg vitamin C)

Vitamin E will ensure that fatty acids are maintained at optimum efficiency once they are absorbed into cells. In addition, vitamin E has anti-inflammatory effects and increases resistance to infection. Use only natural vitamin E (d-alpha-tocopherol), not the synthetic form (dl-alpha-tocopherol). A mixed tocopherol form of vitamin E is best because children need the gamma as well as the alpha forms.

A **calcium** supplement (500 mg) is essential for children who are restricting dairy products. The best forms of calcium for supplementation are calcium malate or calcium citrate; the alternative compound calcium carbonate is not readily absorbed and is produced from oyster shells, which can be contaminated with heavy metals. Magnesium is usually added to calcium supplements to assist in calcium absorption.

Zinc stimulates immune function, prevents infections, and acts as a cofactor in many enzyme reactions, including the creation of antioxidants. Children with allergies and frequent infections should take extra zinc. If zinc supplementation is continued over a prolonged period of time, it should be given in conjunction with copper in a ratio of ten to one to prevent copper deficiency.

CHAPTER 3

Healthy Decisions

Sleeping Arrangements

Newborn infants sleep an average of sixteen hours per day. Sleep time usually decreases over the first year to fourteen hours per day, equivalent to ten hours at night and two hour-long naps during the day. Any parent will tell you, however, that this average varies widely depending on the child. Some toddlers take a forty-five-minute nap in the morning and a three-hour nap in the afternoon. Some children hardly seem to sleep at all. Your child is likely to get all the sleep that she needs, and most children self-regulate their sleep patterns quite well. Babies do wake from sleep to nurse. Many infants will sleep for five hours at a stretch in the night. Others wake every hour or two to nurse. Some 4-month-old babies sleep for long stretches, but by 9 months are waking every hour. All of these patterns are normal.

A problem that parents sometimes encounter is babies who trade night for day, who think that nighttime is a great time for playing. These babies may need some encouragement to sleep less during the day and more at night. Babies who sleep with their parents usually become attuned to parental sleep patterns and learn by example that nighttime is for sleep. I do not recommend that parents allow their babies to cry themselves to sleep or put babies in a separate room to learn how to fall asleep alone. Babies thrive when their needs are met promptly and they have intimate contact with a parent most of the time. Swaddling your baby in a receiving blanket during the first month will also help to prevent frequent night waking and actually increases the amount of total REM sleep during naps or the night (Gerard et al., 2002).

Most babies will fall asleep while nursing, and mothers are able to put them down after a feeding. In the postpartum period for a few weeks mothers should get plenty of rest. Napping with your baby will rejuvenate you and speed your own recovery from the rigors of labor and birthing. Even with older infants, a quick nap with your baby can be refreshing. Unfortunately, this luxury is often only possible with the first baby. A toddler in the house is not likely to allow mom to take a nap unless he is also sleeping. None of these sleep patterns are much in a parent's control, and babies will usually guide the program.

Many mothers choose to keep their infants close to their own bodies during the day in a sling, when the baby is awake and asleep. Babies naturally sleep best next to a parent's body. Wearing your baby in a sling for most activities is optimal, but parents may also want to put their babies down in a bassinet or cradle (or a crib for an older baby) for extended naptimes. You may choose to nurse your baby while lying in bed before a nap, which is perfectly fine, but then you should place your baby in a safe sleeping space when you get up, either the bassinet or crib. An infant is not safe alone in the parents' bed. Babies can become entangled in covers while sleeping unattended or become trapped in the space between the mattress and the bed frame, or between the bed and a wall. Babies can also simply fall out of bed. Use a bed rail (also called a guardrail) in a bed with a mattress and box springs only if your baby is over 1 year of age—infants can become trapped in the space between the mattress and the bed rail. Even for older children, it is safer to roll up a bath or beach towel and stuff it into the space between the bed rail and mattress.

The question that parents must decide is where their baby will sleep at night. There are four options: bassinets, cribs, sidecars, and in the parents' bed. A sidecar is a three-sided bed that attaches to the side of the parents' bed at the same level as the mattress. This arrangement keeps baby within arm's reach, but outside of your space in the bed. It is especially useful for babies who tend to be restless during the night. On the other hand, most parents are happy to cuddle up with their baby and suffer a few elbows or kicks in the middle of the night.

The most natural place for babies during the night is in the parents' bed. If babies are close, then parents will be able to respond quickly to crying or hunger. Why get out of bed to care for a crying baby if you can just turn to him and provide comfort and food? Sharing a bed is the arrangement of choice and quite customary in most of the world. A great deal of evidence shows that bedsharing, or co-sleeping, is beneficial to establish natural biorhythms in infants, to reduce the incidence of Sudden Infant Death Syndrome (SIDS), and to establish strong emotional bonds between parents and babies. The father-infant bond especially benefits from a co-sleeping arrangement. Mothers establish an intimate bond with their babies in the breastfeeding relationship. Nighttime can provide a similar kind of closeness for fathers and babies. Attachment parenting proponents feel that bedsharing leads to confident and self-reliant children. The benefits of bedsharing are plentiful, rewarding, and comforting. Breastfeeding is easier. Everyone tends to sleep better, and children feel safe. Of course, parents can also closely monitor their baby during the night if their baby is lying right next to them.

I recommend that parents sleep with their infant for at least the first three months of life. During this adjustment period babies are learning to physically adapt to the world around them. Evidence suggests that infants actually learn to breathe by sleeping next to their mothers. A fascinating study showed that even placing a mechanical breathing teddy bear next to newborns with breathing interruption during sleep reduces these episodes by 60 percent (Thoman and Graham, 1986). This may explain the reduced incidence of SIDS among babies that sleep with their parents. A study in South Africa showed that bedsharing babies have higher survival rates than solitary-sleeping babies (Kibel and Davies, 2000). Asian countries, where co-sleeping is the norm, have some of the lowest SIDS rates in the world. This is true for Japan, China, Vietnam, Cambodia, Thailand, and Hong Kong (Davies, 1985; Lee et al., 1999; Fukai and Hiroshi, 2000; Yelland et al., 1996; Nelson et al., 2001).

Researchers investigating the nighttime behavior of breastfeeding and bedsharing mothers and infants recorded and evaluated videotapes of the families through the night. They discovered that the typical mother adopted a position with her knees drawn up under the baby's feet and her upper arm positioned above her baby's head. This allows the mother constant control over the baby's movements in the bed, and keeps her close to the baby's body to monitor the baby's temperature and breathing. Mothers of formula-fed babies took a less protective position, sometimes facing away from their babies, and did not sleep curled up around their infants. All babies tended to sleep between the parents. Breastfed babies also spent some time on the outside of the mother to facilitate access to the other breast. Breastfed babies slept on their sides, formula-fed babies slept supine (Richard, 1996).

If you choose to share your bed with your baby, then you will need to consider how long to maintain this arrangement. It is perfectly fine for children to remain in their parents' bed until they want to leave. Sometimes this occurs at 2 years of age, sometimes as late as age 6. While making this decision, you may want to read some of the books devoted to the subject of bedsharing listed in the appendix. The books by pediatricians Jay Gordon and William Sears are especially useful.

The two most common concerns about sharing a bed with your chil-

GUIDELINES FOR SLEEPING WITH YOUR BABY

RECOMMENDATIONS FROM ATTACHMENT PARENTING INTERNATIONAL:

Always place baby to sleep on back.

Baby should sleep next to mother, rather than between mother and father.

Take precautions to prevent baby from rolling out of bed. Use a mesh guardrail and be sure the guardrail is flush against the mattress and fill in any crevice with a rolled-up baby blanket or towel.

Use a large bed with a mattress that fits snugly against the rail or is flush up against a wall. Don't use fluffy bedding or cover baby with comforters, etc.

Do not sleep with your baby if you are under the influence of alcohol, drugs, or sleep-inducing over-the-counter medications, or if you are overly exhausted from sleep deprivation.

Do not allow babysitters or older siblings to sleep with baby.

Don't fall asleep with baby on a couch, beanbag chair, or waterbed.

Do not let baby sleep unattended on an adult bed.

Don't overly bundle baby, because they get additional warmth from the mother's body. Overheating can be dangerous to infants.

dren are fear of rolling onto your baby, and interference with parental intimacy. Neither of these fears is warranted. Mothers do not accidentally smother their babies. An attentive, breastfeeding mother is extraordinarily sensitive to her baby's location and needs. As for sex, infants will sleep through anything. Older children can be moved to an alternative sleeping location while parents steal a few moments alone together, or parents can slip away to another location themselves, or a baby can be temporarily moved off to the other side of the bed with pillows guarding the edge. Be creative, and you can continue a happy bedsharing relationship with your baby and still maintain the intimacy of your marriage.

If you choose to use a crib, you can place it in your bedroom. I do not consider it safe to leave an infant in a separate room during the night. If your baby becomes accustomed to sleeping in a crib, then at some later point you can move the crib to the baby's room. Babies can get trapped between the mattress and bars of a crib, so you must use bumpers on a crib. Each bumper should have at least six ties, and each tie should be no longer than six inches to avoid strangulation.

Other factors besides sleeping alone can contribute to an increased risk of SIDS, which occurs with 82 out of 100,000 babies in the U.S. Other aspects of sleeping arrangements have an influence on SIDS incidence, and a variety of different drugs contribute to infant deaths. SIDS has been associated with sleeping on soft mattresses and allowing babies to sleep on couches or other soft surfaces (beanbag chairs, overstuffed chairs, waterbeds). Sleeping next to an older sibling is not safe for infants. Parents attuned to their baby will wake if a problem occurs. Older siblings could potentially lie on a baby or injure a baby during the night. Infants who sleep in the face-down position have an increased risk of SIDS.

Several drugs contribute to a higher risk of SIDS. Maternal smoking has been implicated in the occurrence of SIDS in many studies (Chong et al., 2004). Alcohol and recreational drug use, sleeping pills and other sedatives taken by mothers have all been associated with SIDS (Carroll-Pankhurst and Mortimer, 2001). Even vaccination has been implicated in the occurrence of SIDS (Neustaedter, 2002).

The other factor that is always present as a risk for SIDS is the bed or crib mattress itself.

Mattress Dangers
Alarming research suggests that the gases emitted from mattresses treated

with various flame-retarding chemicals, including most adult, bassinet, and crib mattresses, may be associated with SIDS. When naturally occurring fungi grow in a mattress, they react with chemical compounds of phosphorus, arsenic, and antimony used as fire retardants, producing a toxic gas cloud that hovers just above the bed. Turning babies onto their backs to sleep has resulted in a dramatic decrease in deaths, because the babies' noses are no longer stuffed into the mattress where the concentration of gases is highest, according to New Zealand researcher James Sprott.

The solution to the problem of toxic gases released from beds is to wrap all mattresses in an impermeable membrane. There are two ways to accomplish this. Buy a BabeSafe mattress cover for a bassinet or crib. You can find these by searching on the Internet for BabeSafe, or go to www.healthychild.com to find adult or crib mattress covers. The second alternative is to buy polyethylene sheeting (at least 5-mil thickness), available at hardware stores, to make your own mattress cover. Since a mattress-wrapping campaign was initiated in 1994 in New Zealand, the rate of SIDS has dropped by 48 percent, and no infants sleeping on mattresses wrapped in polyethylene have died (Sprott, 1996).

A study published in the *British Medical Journal* (Tappin et al., 2002) confirmed other research associating crib mattresses with SIDS. This study sought to examine whether infants who died without obvious cause were more likely to sleep on a used mattress. Dr. Sprott contends that older, used mattresses will contain more fungus growth and release more toxic gas, and the British study lends further credence to Dr. Sprott's findings. This research study in Scotland investigated whether infants who slept on a previously used mattress were more likely to die of SIDS. The researchers reported that routine use of a mattress previously used by another child was significantly associated with greater risk of SIDS. This evidence should reinforce your resolve to wrap your infant's mattress with polyethylene. This includes the bassinet, the crib, or your own mattress if you sleep with your baby.

How to Wrap a Mattress for SIDS Prevention

Wrap any mattress that your baby uses for sleeping, and leave the wrap on until your baby is well past the age of a risk from SIDS (12 months). Here are the steps.

1. Use thick, clear (not colored) polyethylene sheeting, available in the paint section of your local hardware store. The thickness of the polyethylene must be at least 125 microns, or 5 mil. Polyvinylchloride (PVC) should never be used for wrapping mattresses. Measure the mattress and figure enough extra to cover the sides and part of the bottom of the mattress along the entire perimeter. Cut the appropriate size piece for the mattress and air it outdoors for a few days before you wrap the mattress.

2. Covering an adult mattress is a two-person job; you can probably wrap a crib mattress without help. Place the polyethylene over the top of the mattress and down the ends and sides, and then secure it firmly beneath the mattress with strong adhesive or duct tape. The polyethylene should not be airtight on the underside of the mattress, but it must be airtight on the top and sides of the mattress.

3. On top of the polyethylene place a pure cotton blanket or mattress cover and tuck this in securely. Organic mattress covers are available through www.healthychild.com or other sources on the Internet. Then make the bed using pure cotton or pure wool sheets and blankets. Do not use any of the following items in your baby's bed: sheepskin, any form of moisture-resistant mattress protector, or acrylic blanket, sleeping bag, or duvet.

SAFE SLEEP WITH YOUR BABY

Use a firm mattress

Cover all mattresses with polyethylene

Have babies sleep on their back or side

Sleep facing your baby

Do not allow babies to sleep in water beds

Fill all crevices between the mattress and bed frame with foam or pillows

Use bumpers in cribs

Use bed rails for children over age 1

Sleep between an older child and an infant

Drinking Water

Once upon a time it was so simple. Either the water was safe or it outright killed you. Along came chlorine and water became a lot less questionable and life-threatening. Or so we thought. In today's world, with life expectancy in the eighties and beyond, we would like to stay healthy for as long as possible. Long-range effects of toxins become more important, and thus our newfound concern with pesticides, poisoned fish, vaccines, and water. One would think the lowly H_2O molecule would be a no-brainer, as far as safety goes, but alas the water from taps (coming as it does through questionable pipes) and the bottled stuff in stores (coming from multinational corporations) must be scrutinized.

Luckily for us, we only have two choices. Drink it out of the tap or get it from a bottling company, unless you happen to have your own non-

polluted stream (if there were such a thing) or a handy rain barrel. So
for most of us the choice is simple: Take your chances or try to make
what we have as safe as possible.

The first step may be to test your water. This would be advisable if
you live in farm country or have well sources. Be advised though, that
the testing is only good for the day on which the sample was taken. If you
are curious about your tap water, bottled water, or the efficiency of your
filter, you may want to test it too. A quality water testing service is on the
Internet at www.aquamd.com, or AquaMD at 1-866-278-2634. Testing
will determine whether you need to filter your water, with either of
two distinct kinds of filters.

We'll get to the filtering process and types, but first, let's eliminate
one approach that may have been suggested as an alternative. *Do not
drink distilled water.* Distillation may not remove all contaminating chemicals, but it certainly does remove minerals that are essential to health.
The water will then leach minerals from your body, causing deficiencies. This will eventually cause an abnormally acidic environment, which
can lead to serious chronic disease.

Tap Water

The problems with tap water are numerous. This is unavoidable. The
federal government and the EPA set maximum levels of various contaminants in drinking water. Municipalities must conform to these
requirements. If these levels are exceeded, what happens? Nothing. If
people are getting sick, you will be notified to boil your water.

Here are the problems. Chlorine easily reacts with other molecules
to create chlorinated chemicals (chloroform, formaldehyde). Chlorine
by-products from water treatment have been associated with bladder and
rectal cancer. Chlorine in water can also initiate and aggravate allergic
reactions and skin irritation. It also reacts with water-borne decaying

organic matter creating trihalomethanes (THMs), one of which is for-maldehyde, a known carcinogen. Chloramine does not create THMs and has increasingly replaced chlorine as a disinfectant, but greater concentrations need to be used compared to chlorine, and chloramine has been shown to cause similar reactions. It also kills fish if added to a fish tank.

Tap water may be relatively clean when it comes from the processing plant, but it has a long journey through pipes to your house. The pipes, possibly very old, may add lead, asbestos, copper, or PVC breakdown products to your water—all of these are toxic. The pipes may also be decayed and have holes that allow bacteria to proliferate or ground con-taminants (pesticides, arsenic, and other petrochemicals) to seep into the water passing through the pipes. Cysts of protozoa (giardia) can per-sist even in chlorinated water. *Do not drink tap water unless it is filtered. Never give unfiltered tap water to infants.*

What Kind of Filter?

Only one type of filter, a solid carbon block water filter, truly works. Here are the details. The three common types of filters use loose gran-ular activated carbon, reverse osmosis, or solid carbon block.

Carbon absorbs impurities. Activated carbon has a slight electro-positive charge added to it that attracts chemicals and impurities. Loose granular activated carbon filters have a filter like loose sand. This is the most common type of filters one can buy in hardware and discount stores, but it is not an adequate method of water filtration. Bacteria can proliferate within the filter, and much of the water that passes through does not come in contact with the carbon. These filters will not remove chemicals.

Reverse osmosis filters force water through a semi-permeable mem-brane. The membrane blocks minerals, so the water will be mineral-deficient, which in turn will cause mineral deficiencies in those who drink it. Reverse osmosis does not remove chemicals or other contaminants, so a carbon filter is often added.

A solid carbon block filter does what it sounds like—it forces water through a solid block. This prevents channels of water from bypassing the carbon. The technology and construction of solid carbon blocks differ with various companies depending on the density of the block and the nature of the outer membrane surrounding the block. However, consumers can rely on the NSF ratings of these filters. Solid carbon block water filters are the only filters that pass the National Sanitation Foundation (NSF) Standard #53 for health effects. This standard includes removal of chemicals, pesticides, herbicides, cysts, lead, asbestos, and radon. Some filters are now also rated for filtration of the gas additive MTBE. Websites and literature of filter manufacturers should list the substances each filter does remove. Standard #42 rates chlorine removal. Class 1 means 75 percent or greater chlorine removal.

These filters come in different configurations; they can be installed on the counter, under the sink, inline, or as entire house systems.

Solid carbon block filters will not remove nitrates and sulfides (by-products of agricultural fertilization). If you live in an area with extensive farming, you may want to have your water tested for these products. If they are present, then you will need an additional reverse osmosis filter to remove them. Remember that this water is then deficient in minerals, and everyone in the family will need to take a good multi-mineral supplement.

Only buy a carbon block filter that passes the NSF standards #53 and #42. The warranty of these filters should be three to five years. Filters should last for a year with normal use, and consumers should investigate the cost of filter replacement before their purchase.

If your water is fluoridated, then you will need an additional inline filter designed specifically to remove fluoride (for information, go to www.crystalquest.com).

Bottled Water

In reaction to a damning report issued by the Natural Resources Defense Council entitled *Bottled Water: Pure Drink or Pure Hype?*, the International Bottled Water Association replied in their own report that bottled water meets standards for contamination equal to those applied to tap water. This is not very reassuring, given what I have just told you about the hazards of drinking unfiltered tap water. You can find the two reports at these website links:

http://www.nrdc.org/water/drinking/nbw.asp

http://www.bottledwater.org/public/BWFactsHome_main.htm

Bottled water comes from various sources. At least 25 percent of bottled water is actually just bottled tap water. "Purified water" probably means tap water that has been filtered in some fashion. Many bottles labeled "spring water" come from underground wells or aquifers that may be in close proximity to industrial sites. A call to your bottled water provider will tell you where the water comes from and may reassure you, but it will not tell you what is in your water no matter what their testing reports say. Our vision of bottled water is crystal-pure mountain snows and glaciers delivered in their pristine state for your pleasure and delectation. The bottled water industry encourages this utopian vision, even as they defend against lawsuits charging misrepresentation of the sources of "spring" water.

Bottled water also suffers from other problems. Although it is not run to your house through old, decaying pipes, it is packaged in plastic. Most clear plastic bottles seem to be safe, especially those labeled 1, 2, and 4. However, water that is delivered in five-gallon polycarbonate bottles (number 7) that have been reused may leach bisphenol A (BPA) into the water. The plastics industry insists that bottles do not leach BPA and that BPA does not cause problems (see www.plasticsinfo.org). Others would differ, since BPA has been linked to chromosome damage and hormone disruption (see page 22). Limitation of our exposure to estrogenic plastics seems essential because of the carcinogenic nature of estrogen. Whether we get significant amounts of these xenoestrogens from water bottles remains unclear. If we do, then children would be especially at risk.

Plastic bottles also have a significant impact on the environment. Even if they are recycled, energy must be used to remold them into new bottles.

The water cooler represents another potential reservoir for contaminants when considering delivered bottled water. Running boiling water through your water cooler once a month will help prevent the buildup of bacteria and algae. Use a pottery water cooler, not one with a plastic container.

Summary

Filter all tap water for drinking through a solid carbon block filter. Change the filter as advised by the manufacturer. If you use bottled water, do some investigation about the source of the water that you buy. Clean the water cooler with boiling water periodically. Do not reuse plastic bottles because of the danger of bacterial contamination and the possible leaching of plastics after washing with detergents.

Water Bottles

Bottled water is here to stay—this is a booming industry that grosses more than $7 billion a year in the U.S. Water is good, and we know that hydration is essential, especially when children are exercising and playing sports. But the bottles your children are drinking water from may be dangerous to their health.

Polycarbonate water bottles (labeled #7) contain bisphenol A (BPA), which leaches from the plastic even at room temperature and has been linked to chromosome damage and hormone disruption. These are the types of plastic Nalgene water bottles found in sports stores. The genetic damage caused by BPA from polycarbonate plastic was discovered by accident. Plastic mice cages were washed with a harsh detergent and the female mice were subsequently found to have abnormal cell division in their oocytes (the immature ovarian cells that develop into eggs). The abnormality was traced to the BPA, and the exposure was reproduced in an intentional laboratory study (Hunt et al., 2003). A follow-up study determined that new and used polycarbonate animal cages released BPA with estrogenic properties into water when the cages were kept at room temperature (Kembra et al., 2003).

#1 PET or PETE bottles (polyethylene terephthalate) may leach DEHA, a known carcinogen, if used more than once. Additionally, your water bottle that has been refilled is likely to contain potentially harmful bacteria that grow on saliva, food particles, and fecal material from unwashed hands. Many people have reported getting diarrhea from their reused water bottles. Washing bottles with hot water and detergent or a rinse with bleach will sanitize them, but also leaches harmful chemicals out of the plastic.

What to Do?

Use metal bottles. A Swiss company, SIGG, makes colorful and safe aluminum drinking bottles lined with an impermeable alloy. They can be found on the Internet and at many specialty sports stores. They offer both children's and adult's sizes and designs. Many other sites carry SIGG bottles as well. Thermos makes stainless steel bottles for both hot and

---

PLASTIC CONTAINERS

RELATIVELY SAFE:

> #1 polyethylene terephthalate (PET), used only once

> #2 and #4 polyethylene

UNSAFE:

> #5 polypropylene (catsup bottles, yogurt containers)

> #6 polystyrene (Styrofoam)

> #7 polycarbonate (Nalgene) water bottles

NEVER USE:

> Food or drinks heated in plastic containers in a microwave

> Styrofoam cups (#6 polystyrene) for hot liquids

> #7 polycarbonate (Nalgene) water bottles

> Plastic baby bottles (If you must use bottles, use glass baby bottles with silicone, not latex, nipples.)

---

cold drinks or soups; they are available at www.thermos.com. Other companies also make stainless steel water bottles; check out www.kleankanteen.com. Wash these bottles and their tops with hot water by hand after use. Dishwashers may not get into the narrow mouths of water bottles to clean their interiors, so wash them with a bottle brush.

Safer plastic containers are high-density #2 polyethylene and low-density #4 polyethylene (HDPE #2 and LDPE #4). HDPE is used for milk, water, juice, and yogurt containers. LDPE is used for squeezable bottles (honey, mustard, etc.).

Buy food products packaged in glass whenever possible. Use glass containers for storing leftovers. Do not reuse plastic water bottles. Throw away plastic sippy cups after prolonged use and buy new ones.

And don't forget to have children wash their hands after using the bathroom.

Shampoos, Lotions, and Powders

Your child's skin absorbs chemicals very efficiently. Skin patches are an excellent way to administer drugs because they will then bypass the digestive system, avoiding unwanted side effects. The skin absorbs many substances more reliably than the digestive tract. Be careful what you put on your child's skin. Read labels on shampoo and skin care products and you will discover a new world of exotic chemicals. The products that touch your baby's skin include wipes, diaper rash creams, shampoo, soap, and moisturizers. Powders are not appropriate for babies. Talc is composed of sharp, fine particles that can irritate a baby's airways. Even cornstarch can be an irritant to airways when inhaled. Avoid using powder on your baby. Choose baby wipes that do not contain alcohol. Seventh Generation Baby Wipes and Tushies Wipes contain only natural ingredients, without alcohol.

Shampoo

Of all the baby care products, shampoos tend to have the most ingredients. Use a shampoo that has natural herbal ingredients, preferably organic. Products by Aubrey Organics, California Baby, Dr. Bronner, and others are safer than commercial shampoos. Two of the most problematic ingredients in shampoo are sodium lauryl sulfate (SLS) and propylene glycol. SLS is a wetting and foaming agent frequently used in shampoos and toothpastes. It can cause skin irritation, mucous mem-

CHEMICALS TO AVOID IN SHAMPOO

Sodium lauryl (or laureth) sulfate

Propylene glycol

Polyethylene glycol (PEG)

Ethanolamines (DEA, MEA, TEA)

Alcohol

Fragrance

Parabens (methyl-, propyl-, ethyl-)

brane irritation, urinary tract infections, and drying of the skin, and it is
a mutagen capable of causing changes in genetic material in cells. Propylene glycol is a wetting agent or solvent. It is a common component of
anti-freeze and brake fluid. It has been linked with kidney damage and
liver abnormalities as well as rashes and dry skin.

Other common ingredients are not much better. Polyethylene glycol
(PEG) is a degreaser used in spray-on oven cleaners. PEG dries the skin
and has been identified as a potential carcinogen. DEA, MEA, and TEA,
the ethanolamines, are hormone-disrupting chemicals used in dry cleaning fluids and paint; they are known to form cancer-causing nitrates
and nitrosamines. These foaming agents have been associated with liver
and kidney cancer. The synthetic paraben preservatives methyl-, ethyl-
and propylparaben are also hormone disrupters with toxic properties.
Some preservatives (urea and DMDM hydantoin) added to skin and
hair products release formaldehyde. The word "fragrance" denotes synthetic compounds with up to 4,000 separate ingredients, many of which

are carcinogenic, toxic, and capable of producing a wide range of symptoms including hyperactivity, irritability, headaches, and skin irritation. See page 22 for a discussion of hormone disruption.

Lotions and Creams

Some excellent products exist for moisturizing and protecting your baby's skin. Products with essential oils can be especially soothing. Avoid lotions, ointments, and creams that contain petroleum or petrolatum and alcohol. Many of the same harmful chemicals found in shampoos will also show up in lotions. Companies that make an effort to use only natural ingredients include Weleda, Mustela, and California Baby. Each makes diaper creams and baby lotions that are soothing and nontoxic.

Chlorine

The water you use to wash your baby is treated with chlorine. If your home has a full-house filter, it will remove chlorine. Otherwise you can purchase a showerhead chlorine filter and use a bath ball that hangs under the tub faucet. They will remove up to 100 percent of chlorine from the water using copper and zinc (KDF) to convert chlorine to harmless zinc chloride. Chloramine is similarly removed from tub bath water when the chlorine is liberated from the chlorine-ammonia bond and converted to a zinc chloride salt. Another alternative is to add vitamin C chlorine removal tablets to the bathwater. You can search on the Internet for product sources, using these headings: chlorine bath ball, shower filter, dechlorinating bath tabs.

Skin exposure to chlorine causes a number of potential health problems. Chlorinated water is a skin irritant that destroys essential fatty acids and vitamin E while generating toxins capable of free-radical damage. Chlorine causes rashes and aggravates eczema. Swimming in chlorinated pools aggravates asthma (Mustchin and Pickering, 1979; AAAI,

2001). The skin absorbs more chlorine during a ten-minute shower than from from drinking eight glasses of chlorinated water.

Trihalomethanes (THMs) are carcinogens formed by chlorine's interaction with organic compounds in water. During showers THMs and chlorine are released as vapors and easily inhaled. It is estimated that household members can receive six to 100 times more chlorine by breathing the air around showers than they would from drinking the water (Anderson, 1986). The amount of chlorine inhaled from one shower is equivalent to drinking two liters of water. For a discussion of the hazards of chlorine and other components of drinking water, see page 66.

Replacing showerheads with shower filters and removing chlorine from children's baths with a ball for the faucet or dechlorinating tablets can eliminate all of the potentially toxic effects of chlorine in baths and showers.

Environmental Toxins

You can take many simple steps to limit your child's exposure to household environmental toxins. Never use drain cleaners made from lye or oven cleaners that release toxic gases. Use only non-chlorine scouring powders (Bon Ami brand). Baking soda also works well to clean sinks and tubs. Avoid spray cleaners, conventional detergents, disinfectants, and bleach cleaners. Use cleaning products made by environmentally friendly companies that use nontoxic ingredients (Seventh Generation, Ecover, and Aubrey Organics). Use mineral oil instead of furniture polish that contains solvents. Use a vinegar and water solution on windows, TV screens, and computer monitors instead of glass cleaners that contain ammonia. You may need to wipe the glass with alcohol first to remove the wax from previous glass cleaners. Both aerosol and solid air fresheners typically contain carcinogenic compounds that are dispersed into

---

ENVIRONMENTAL TOXINS IN THE HOME

Oven cleaners	Drain cleaners
Chlorine scouring powders	Commercial glass cleaners
Toxic paints	Air fresheners
Weed killers	Bug sprays

---

the home. Common ingredients include formaldehyde, benzene, and synthetic fragrances produced from petroleum distillates capable of causing cancer, birth defects, central nervous system disorders, and allergic reactions (National Academy of Sciences, 1986). Use nontoxic latex and enamel paint when painting your home. Use nontoxic products for construction and decorating (floors, carpets, furniture) from sources like www.healthyhomedesigns.com and www.greenbuildingsupply.com.

Never use pesticide chemicals in your home. If you have a continuing problem with pests, then use only Integrated Pest Management (IPM) strategies. You can find these resources on the Internet IPM strategies will provide nontoxic solutions to most pest infestations of insects, mites, or rodents. Some of these strategies may include the use of boric acid or diatomaceous earth to kill fleas and heat treatments to eliminate termites. Check the website www.beyondpesticides.org for more information about keeping your home environment pesticide-free.

Never use herbicides or weed killers around your house. They are not safe for children. For example, Roundup weed killer has been linked to attention problems in children, Parkinson's disease, and cancer. At least two studies have demonstrated an association between Roundup (glyphosate) and non-Hodgkin's lymphoma, a deadly form of lymph system cancer (Hardell and Eriksson, 1999). An article in the journal

Soil and Health reported that two studies failed to confirm the U.S. EPA's classification of glyphosate as non-carcinogenic (Watts, 1998). Similarly, the use of pesticides in and around the home has been associated with childhood leukemia, sarcoma, and brain tumors. Prenatal exposure is especially harmful. These poisons also drastically alter hormone development in children (see page 22).

Plastic Toys and Phthalates

Are your child's toys safe? Do you ever wonder whether your baby should chew on a plastic toy? Most of the toys you have in the house are made of polyvinylchloride (PVC), which is a hard, brittle plastic. In order to make PVC softer, squishier, and squeezable, manufacturers add one or more of the various phthalates (pronounced thalates). These phthalates are not chemically bound to the PVC molecules. They sit alongside them and easily leach out of the toys when sucked, chewed, or heated (left in the sun). That new-car smell is phthalates leaching from your car's dashboard into the air. Perfumes, deodorants, hair products, plastic wrap, and lotions also contain phthalates. If a product's ingredient list includes the word "fragrance," it most likely contains phthalates.

Phthalates are toxic. They cause cancer, kidney damage, and decreased sperm production in rats (Agency for Toxic Substances, 1993). Phthalates are estrogenic hormone disruptors. They have been identified as a possible cause of premature breast development in young girls (Colon et al., 2000). Men exposed to background environmental levels of phthalates have shown DNA damage to sperm (Duty et al., 2003) and abnormal sperm motility and sperm concentration (Duty et al., 2003a).

Here is what you can do. Buy toys made of wood, metal, or cloth. Buy plastic toys labeled #2 or #4 (polyethylene). Toys that are not labeled probably contain PVC and phthalates. Choose unscented personal care

---

SOURCES OF PHTHALATE EXPOSURE IN THE HOME

Soft plastic toys	Perfumes and fragrances
Hair products	Deodorants
Lotions	Plastic wrap

---

products and avoid the word "fragrance." Use products labeled organic and scented only with essential oils. Some companies have chosen not to use phthalates (Aubrey Organics, Avalon, Jason, Kiss My Face, Logona, Nature's Gate, Tom's of Maine, Weleda, and others). Many of these products can be found at your local health food store or online.

Drugs and Medications

What factors in your child's life are most likely to cause health problems? First, of course, are genetic factors, such as a tendency to develop allergies. You can minimize the effect of genetic tendencies by maintaining excellent health and nutrition during pregnancy and while breastfeeding. A second factor is exposure to drugs and medications, and this is an area where personal choice is important. You can choose whether your child gets drugs and medications, and which ones your child gets.

The first class of drugs your child will use is **vaccines**. These are by far the most potent drugs your child is likely to take. They are capable of inflicting damage to nerves and the brain, resulting in permanent problems including autism, learning disorders, and seizures. They can also damage the immune system, causing asthma, diabetes, and immune deficiency states that result in a susceptibility to recurrent colds and ear infections. (See page 85 for a more thorough discussion of vaccines.)

The next class of drugs is **antibiotics**, which may result in a quick fix for some types of infections, but can damage the delicate balance of immune functions in children and cause recurrences of the very same infections they are intended to treat.

Then there are the **suppressive**, or symptom-reduction, drugs: decongestants, antihistamines, cough medicines, pain relievers, and fever reducers. Many of these have been taken off the market because of dangerous side effects. A study published in *Pediatrics* proves that cough syrups have no effect on children's coughs (Paul et al., 2004). And they are dangerous. (See page 227 for more about coughs.) The fever reducers now contain a warning label about their side effects, and such warnings may be downplaying the damaging effects of these over-the-counter drugs on the nervous system. (For more discussion of fever treatment, see page 235.)

Finally, there are the **chemicals** added to packaged foods and drinks. Children should never ingest aspartame (Nutrasweet) or monosodium glutamate (MSG). These substances, known as excitotoxins, have significant negative effects on nervous system functions. Other added chemicals are hidden in terms such as "textured vegetable protein" and "natural and artificial flavorings."

Sun and Sunscreen

You are concerned about cumulative damage to your child's skin from sun exposure, so you use a sunscreen. But what about those strange-sounding chemicals. Are they safe? The answer is no. Most sunscreens contain a mixture of some of the following ingredients: oxybenzone, methoxycinnamate, salicylates, PABA, benzophenones, benzoylmethanes, and triethanolamine. These toxic chemicals are absorbed through

SAFETY OF ZINC OXIDE AND TITANIUM DIOXIDE SUNSCREENS

ZINC OXIDE:

According to OSHA, topical administration of zinc oxide to rabbits, mice, and guinea pigs failed to cause either skin irritation or signs of systemic toxicity (ACGIH, 1991).

TITANIUM DIOXIDE:

Titanium dioxide is not toxic, according to the EPA's toxicological profile:

Titanium is the eighth most abundant element in the earth's crust and consequently spontaneously enters the food chain to some degree. Titanium dioxide (TiO_2) is a major constituent of a number of minerals, including rutile, which consists of 95% titanium dioxide. The most commercially important of the titanium compounds, titanium dioxide annual worldwide production is estimated to be appoximately two million metric tons. Titanium dioxide is an opaque powder that is approved for use as a colorant in food (21 CFR 73.575), in drugs (21 CFR 73.1575), and in cosmetics (21 CFR 73.2575; 21 CFR 73.3126). It has an extensive range of industrial uses (e.g., paint, paper, and plastics). Titanium dioxide is currently exempt from the requirement for a tolerance when used as a colorant in pesticide formulations (40 CFR 180.1001(d)). A National Cancer Institute bioassay concluded that titanium dioxide did not affect mortality, and was not carcinogenic at dose levels of 25,000 or 50,000 ppm in rats or mice. The World Health Organization Committee on Food Coloring Materials has determined that no ADI need be set for the use of titanium dioxide based on the range of acute, subacute and chronic toxicity assays, all showing low mammalian toxicity, including a two year chronic feeding study in mice which was negative for carcinogenicity. Indeed, titanium dioxide is frequently used as a negative control material in in vivo chronic dust exposure studies and in in vivo assessments of fibrogenic potential of dusts.

the skin, and they can cause cancer. Some ingredients, such as cinnamates and salicylates, are also hormone disruptors. Sunscreen ingredients and their metabolites are readily observable in plasma and urine samples after usage by humans (Sarveiya, 2004). They have never been proven safe, and children may be especially susceptible to their harmful effects.

A better solution is to use the sunblockers zinc oxide and titanium dioxide. You can buy these in creams and rub-on sticks at health food stores. A powdered version is also available from ColoreScience in a brush-on form. For children I recommend using only sunscreens with these natural ingredients. Baby and children's sunscreen by Lavera is organic and has an excellent waterproof consistency. Other sources include Aveda, Aubrey Organics, Weleda, and Dr. Hauschka products.

Older children can begin wearing UV protective sunglasses to prevent cataracts later in life, and use sunscreens judiciously. Babies and young children can wear hats to protect them from bright sunlight. Children need sun exposure during the summer months. The vitamin D derived from the interaction of ultraviolet light and their skin will stimulate bone growth, prevent immune system weakness, and protect them from osteoporosis, autoimmune disease, and skin cancer, including melanoma (see page 36). However, it is important to avoid sunburn that can damage your child's skin.

Begin with gradual exposure and limit outdoor play during the time of greatest sun brightness, 10 AM to 2 PM. This will allow gradual development of tanning and avoid burns. If you are out in the hot sun on a tropical beach, or if your child is playing baseball, tennis, or soccer in the hot sun, avoid sunburn by using a sunscreen. Put sunscreen on kids' faces and shoulders when they are spending an afternoon in the pool.

Fluoride

The two important questions about fluoride—questions that should be applied to any drug, medication, or chemical additive—are "Does it work?" and "Is it safe?" According to the FDA, fluoride is an unapproved new drug for which there is no proof of safety or effectiveness. In four major studies involving 480,000 children comparing fluoridated and unfluoridated areas around the world, no significant differences could be found in tooth decay rates. In Western Europe, most countries do not fluoridate their water. A survey using dental examinations found that unfluoridated areas experienced a similar decline in dental caries when compared to fluoridated areas in European countries over a ten-year period (Diesendorf, 1986). In the U.S., the Centers for Disease Control (CDC) points to the decline in dental caries during the period 1970–2000 as proof that fluoridated water reduces the incidence of cavities, but nearly every country in Europe experienced a similar decline in cavities over the same period (Fomon et al., 2000). Similarly, within the U.S., areas with fluoridated water have nearly identical decay rates as unfluoridated areas (Hileman, 1989). Ironically, a U.S. government journal, *Environmental Health Perspectives*, published a study that showed that children in fluoridated Boston had significantly more tooth decay than children living in unfluoridated Farmington, Maine. The problem was traced to the tendency of silicofluorides added to water supplies to increase blood lead level, which in turn is linked to cavities (Gemmel et al., 2002).

Flouride toxicity is well documented. Fluoride causes cancer in rats, and exposure to fluoridated drinking water has been associated with bone cancer in humans (Cohn, 1992). Fluoride exposure causes osteoporosis and increases the risk of hip fractures. In one study, children exposed to fluoride had lower IQ scores, apparently because of fluoride's neurotoxic effects (Li et al., 1995). It causes mottling of tooth enamel. According to the American Dental Association, dentists make 17 percent more profit in fluoridated areas than in unfluoridated areas (Douglas, 1972). Fluoride has a toxicity rating higher than lead.

If you would like to know how an extremely hazardous by-product of metal processing and the fertilizer industry was foisted on the American public by a handful of corporate executives and government bureaucrats, read Christopher Bryson's book *The Fluoride Deception* (Seven Stories Press, 2004).

Do not expose your children to fluoride. Do not use fluoridated toothpaste or fluoride supplements. Do not drink fluoridated water. And do not allow fluoride treatments at the dentist's office. Just say no to fluoride.

CHAPTER 4

The Vaccine Controversy

What Is the Problem with Vaccines?

It is time for the two-month well-baby visit at the pediatrician's office. Your healthy baby is beginning to smile and coo, breastfeeding is finally going well, and you are feeling like proud parents. Then the doctor says it's time for the baby's shots, and she rattles off a list of six diseases with barely recognizable names. Are all of these vaccines necessary? Why so many at once? Are there any side effects? The brochures you receive are overwhelming, but they minimize the side effects, and the doctor insists the shots will prevent deadly diseases. Do you simply go along with the program? Maybe you have heard about bad reactions to vaccines, and you have some apprehension. The needle is poised. What is your decision?

Like most parents, you may feel poorly informed about this medical issue, and so you leave this decision to the doctor. Your pediatrician must have your baby's best interests in mind. Or is there another side to the immunization decision? This is a choice that could affect your child for the rest of his or her life. We are trained to accept doctors' recommendations without question, but wouldn't it be wiser to approach this decision like any other consumer issue and read enough about it to make an informed choice?

Ask the parents who regret not being well informed, the parents

whose children were seriously injured by vaccines. Internet sites overflow with the sorrowful accounts of children maimed or killed by immu-
nizations. The stories ring with the sharp tones of betrayal and tragic
loss. Parents ask why they weren't told that their healthy, happy, normal baby could die from a vaccine. They are further enraged when their
concerns about a relationship between the recently administered vaccine and their child's symptoms are denied by their doctor, the drug
manufacturer, and the government. These authorities usually claim that
the onset of symptoms after a shot is pure coincidence.

What are parents doing about this? They are forming advocacy groups
and confronting what they see as coercive medical laws that force vaccinations on their children—vaccinations that may be dangerous or
unnecessary. One of these parents had the power to make a difference.
When a vaccine apparently injured two of Congressman Dan Burton's
grandchildren, he demanded some accountability. The result was con-
gressional hearings, which began in August 1999 to investigate the cul-
pability of the hepatitis vaccine and a vaccine industry that may be
spinning out of control. During these hearings, representatives asked
some hard-hitting questions: Why target children for a sexually transmitted disease? Why risk the serious adverse reactions associated with this
vaccine? Is the profit motive fueling the vaccine campaign?

Revenues from vaccines total more than $1 billion in the United
States, and $3 billion worldwide. It is expected that this figure will
increase to $7 billion in the next few years. To ensure continuing prof-
its, vaccine manufacturers conduct their own research, pay for ad cam-
paigns encouraging parents to get the shots, and foot the bill for state
legislation to mandate each vaccine for every child in America. Drug
companies enjoy a guaranteed market for their product. After all, in
many states parents are threatened with imprisonment or removal of
their child from their home if they refuse.

Some people point a vigorous accusatory finger at vaccine manufacturers, charging that these companies conveniently bypass the usual checks and balances of the medical and legal systems. Why are vaccine-related adverse events hidden from parents, buried in the medical literature or in obscure reporting systems? Who is making policy decisions? Who is looking out for the health of our children? Doctors employed by drug companies also advise government recommendation panels. The same doctors who are paid consultants for the drug companies that make the product write position papers for the American Academy of Pediatrics. Conflict of interest? Business as usual in the world of vaccines.

Your pediatrician is discouraged from questioning vaccine utilization. Liability issues, boards of medical examiners, and policies of HMOs govern the doctors' recommendations. Step outside this set of rules and they risk their jobs or their licenses. Pediatricians are trained in the benefits and absolute necessity of vaccines; they too are shielded from the reports of adverse effects. Thus, they are insistent that parents vaccinate their children. It is not uncommon for pediatricians to refuse to continue care for a child when parents decline a vaccine. Can you question the pediatrician's advice? Remember, you have hired the pediatrician's services and you are the guardian of your child's health. You will live with the consequences of your decision.

You carefully research other consumer issues. You spend significant amounts of time studying what car to buy, analyzing statistics, safety issues, gas mileage, performance, features, and option packages. You owe it to your baby's future health to do the same research on vaccines that you purchase from a medical provider. Read guides that discuss the diseases—their prevalence in your area, their transmission, their complications. Read about vaccine effectiveness for those diseases, adverse reactions to the vaccines, the chemical components of vaccine formulations, and the alternatives to vaccination. Then make your decision.

What Adverse Reactions Are Possible?

Children suffer two types of adverse events after vaccines. One is an acute, short-lived set of symptoms that culminates in recovery or death. This category includes allergic reactions, nervous system disorders such as paralysis or seizures, arthritis, and a whole range of minor reactions including fevers and swelling at the injection site. In recent years concerns have increased about the second category of adverse reactions, the chronic and unremitting problems that sometimes occur following vaccines. An association with asthma following vaccination, as well as studies showing a connection between vaccines and diabetes and autism, have raised alarm bells among consumers. If vaccines are capable of causing such long-range problems, then perhaps our strategies for disease prevention require re-evaluation. Could these chronic diseases be the result of the bombardment of the infant's immature immune system by the repeated assault of bacterial and viral toxins mixed with chemical additives contained in the routine shots given at the doctor's office?

If vaccines are causing the dramatic increase in childhood asthma, diabetes, and autism, then the cost of vaccination is much higher than we are led to believe. We may be replacing acute infectious diseases with chronic, debilitating, and lifelong illness.

Do Vaccines Work?

The answer may seem obvious and the question heretical to any person raised in the world of modern medicine. The vaccine industry and medical textbooks inform us that immunization is the greatest miracle of preventive medicine.

Some vaccines are more effective in preventing disease than others. The protective effect of the whooping cough vaccine varies dramatically from study to study. The fact that a disease has declined in the population is not proof that the vaccine works. The incidence of many infectious diseases was already declining prior to the use of vaccines. Between 1900 and 1920 the mortality rate from diphtheria decreased by 50 percent, prior to the widespread use of the vaccine and prior to the invention of antibiotics. When vaccines are introduced, statistics are sometimes manipulated to artificially decrease the number of reported cases for a disease. During the polio epidemic of the 1950s, the criteria of diagnosis for paralytic polio were drastically altered after the vaccine was introduced so that the number of reported cases was guaranteed to fall. When the whooping cough vaccine became widely distributed, physicians tended to stop diagnosing whooping cough in their patients, again giving the appearance of a reduction in the number of cases. It is estimated that only 10 percent of whooping cough cases are ever diagnosed. This creates the illusion of effectiveness.

Making an Informed Choice

Become informed about the issues surrounding vaccines. Read books, visit websites. Become a sophisticated and informed consumer. This could be the most important decision you make for your child's health. In order to make an informed decision about vaccination, you need to obtain information. Then you can base your decisions on reasoned and considered thoughts, rather than on the emotional pulls of anxiety about diseases, guilt over challenging accepted views, or fear of outside pressure from family, doctors, or schools.

We are moving away from a fear of isolated diseases toward a view of the body as an entire organism. We now think in terms of the body's immune system strength and its ability to maintain health. The dramatic increase in immune system disorders has led many health care providers

FACTORS TO CONSIDER ABOUT INDIVIDUAL DISEASES

Disease incidence and the likelihood of exposure

Severity and possible complications of the disease

The risks from the disease, compared with the risks from the vaccine

and consumer advocates to question the role of chemical exposure and medical interventions, including vaccines, as a cause of immune system failure. The coincident emergence of immune system disorders (AIDS, lupus, chronic fatigue syndrome, fibromyalgia, MS, and diabetes) with the mass vaccination of populations has led to suspicions that an entire generation has suffered immune system crippling from the vaccines that should be protecting us from illness.

Learn about the diseases and the vaccines, weigh the potential risks yourself. If you are considering vaccinations for your child, then you should know exactly what you are trying to prevent, and why. All vaccines have potential side effects. Before you decide to take the risk of adverse reactions to vaccines in your child, you should know the facts.

Decide which vaccines you do or don't want. You may decide that some are prudent and others are unnecessary for your child. For example, if there is no possibility of your child being exposed to a disease (say, polio or hepatitis B), then it may not make sense for you to risk an adverse reaction to its vaccine. Or if a disease is so mild that complications are extremely unlikely (chicken pox), then lifelong immunity from acquiring the disease naturally may be a better choice than getting the vaccine. Other vaccines may seem sensible to you based on your research, your lifestyle, and your philosophy.

CONTROVERSIAL VACCINES

VACCINES WITH HIGH TOXICITY:	DISEASES WITH LOW INCIDENCE OR SEVERITY:
Pertussis	Chicken pox
Measles	Hepatitis B
Mumps	Diphtheria
Rubella	Polio

If you decide to vaccinate, then choose the right time for the shots. The recommended schedule may not be optimal for your child. Delaying vaccines has been associated with less serious adverse reactions.

The appendix to this book contains references to information about vaccines—books that will help you make an informed decision, and websites that will provide you with research and informative articles—to support your decision-making process.

Vaccine Exemptions

Schools may tell you that your child will not be admitted without vaccines, but all states allow exemptions to vaccination. Nearly half the states allow a philosophical exemption, which means that parents can choose not to give vaccines based on their personal beliefs. All states except Mississippi allow a religious exemption. Obtain a copy of your state's immunization law from your State Health Department and read the requirements. A religious exemption should be worded to conform to the language of the law. Several attorneys specialize in this area, and they can help you obtain a religious exemption.

TB Test

Although a test for tuberculosis is not a vaccine, I have included it in this chapter because it represents an intervention, albeit a diagnostic test, that is similarly presented as a benign, protective necessity. However, TB tests may not be as benign as purported. A TB skin test, the Mantoux (tuberculin) test or the Tine test, involves injecting a small amount of tuberculosis antigen into the skin. A clinician then observes the skin reaction to this test. If there is a positive reaction of swelling, redness, or blistering, then the test is pronounced positive. A positive result means that the person has been exposed to tuberculosis bacteria at some time in the past and has developed antibodies. However, false positive and false negative test results are common. If someone had a TB vaccination at any time in the past, or if they were exposed to TB, then their antibodies to the vaccine will cause a positive TB skin test. Ninety percent of people exposed to TB will not contract the disease. The skin test fails to detect half of people with latent TB, and false-negatives are common in individuals with weakened immune systems. Usually, anyone with a positive skin test for TB is advised to complete at least six months of treatment with the antibiotic isoniazid (INH). It is estimated that 50 percent of people prescribed antibiotics on the basis of a positive skin reaction do not have TB infection at all.

The injection of a small quantity of antigen is not supposed to cause any systemic reaction, but it is possible that even this small amount of TB antigen could trigger the body's immune system to react abnormally. I have seen autoimmune disease processes begin soon after TB tests, and others have also reported this occurrence. This observation does not prove that a TB test can cause this reaction, but it should give us pause before allowing the test to be performed on children.

A much safer, more accurate, quicker, and convenient blood test exists for the detection of tuberculosis infection. The blood test is performed on a plasma sample with results available in twenty-four hours. In Europe the blood test was approved for use in 2004 and will replace the tuberculin skin test. This test is approved to detect both active and latent TB in infants, children, and adults. The test detects T-cell response to infection which can exist in the body for years without symptoms. The population of latently infected people acts as a reservoir of TB with undetected individuals capable of spreading infection. Once the blood test for TB is approved for use in the U.S., then the skin test will be relegated to history.

PART TWO

FROM BIRTH THROUGH EARLY CHILDHOOD

CHAPTER 5

Baby Is Born

New Life

The first hours following a child's birth are remarkable. Your baby is born gasping for air and faced with a new world. Within a short time she adapts, bonds to her parents, and learns to breathe the air and find her sustenance at the breast. Both you and your baby are filled with wonder and, at the same time, confronting this new experience with apprehension.

Parents discover the miracle of creation and the awesome responsibility of caring for this new being. Waves of emotion buffet you in these first hours after birth. Enjoy and remember the enormity of this event. It is a time of raw experience. Inevitably, your first hours and days as a parent will contain a range of emotions. You will feel overwhelmed at the importance of this event and the task ahead, relieved that the birth is completed, worried whether your baby is healthy, and proud of your achievement. Many parents also have difficulty connecting at first to this squirming, frowning creature. The bonds of love connecting you and your baby may take a while to form, but they will, and they will last a lifetime.

The First Moments of Life

What happens in the first few moments after birth? Your birth attendant will suction fluids from your baby's nose and mouth, preparing a clear airway for the first breath. Your baby will be held by the birth attendant either on the bed or delivery table or placed on mom's belly until breathing is established. The first breath may occur immediately after your baby emerges into the world, or it may take a few minutes and some stimulation of the skin to initiate breathing. The baby is still receiving oxygen-rich blood through the umbilical cord. Allowing the cord to feed the baby blood until it stops pulsating will provide an extra margin of safety for your baby's health. The cord blood is rich in red blood cells that provide iron stores to your baby that will persist for the first six months of life. In addition, you should consider storing your baby's cord blood with a cord blood bank in case the blood cells within it are ever needed in the future to treat an illness in child or mother. These immature blood cells, or stem cells, are able to change and mature into any kind of blood cell. Storing them in a specialized facility could provide your family with life-saving treatment if a serious disease ever occurs (heart disease, nerve or brain damage, strokes, or cancer). On the Internet, visit www.parentsguidecordblood.com for a guide to these services and lists of banks, or go to the oldest of these storage facilities, www.cordblood.com, for complete information and pricing. These services need to be arranged prior to the birth.

Once your baby is breathing, she is covered with a small blanket and placed in mom's arms. Holding and touching your baby provides the first loving contact and reassurance that everything is fine. This is life's most significant transition, and everyone needs a time of quiet reflection and recovery. Get to know your baby. Stare into her eyes. Cherish this moment of imprinting. Your baby may be a little groggy if mom had

		APGAR SCORING			
SCORE	HEART RATE	RESPIRATORY EFFORT	REFLEXES	MUSCLE TONE	COLOR
2	100-140	Normal cry	Normal	Good	Pink
1	100	Irregular/shallow	Depressed	Fair	Fair
0	No beat	Apnea for more than 60 seconds	Absent	Flaccid	Bluish

an anesthetic or epidural. If a cesarean section was necessary, then dad or your birth partner can hold and talk to the baby while the doctor is attending to the mother. The familiar and soothing sound of your voice will help orient your baby to these new surroundings. Babies in the uterus do hear sounds and voices. The inner ear is fully functional after five months of fetal development, so your baby already knows your voice at birth. Newborns already prefer the sound of their mother's and father's voice to that of strangers. This preference shows the high degree of mental development evident in your baby even at this young age.

When the cord stops beating, the birth attendant will cut it, allowing mom to put the baby to her breast.

During this flurry of activity, a cursory exam will reveal the baby's sex and any anatomic abnormalities that may have gone unnoticed at the ultrasounds during pregnancy. Vital signs are recorded at one minute after birth and again at five minutes. These signs include heart rate, breathing effort, muscle tone, reflexes, and color. A score of 0, 1, or 2 is assigned to each of these five signs (see the box). The score is used to determine if your baby might need further evaluation or medical care. However, it is usually obvious when babies are distressed following birth and need immediate medical assistance. The score (called the Apgar and named for its inventor) has little significance and does not correlate well with subsequent health problems that are associated with decreased oxygen supply to the baby's brain. It is not a score of your baby's state of health. However, midwives and doctors still commonly use it to keep a record of the baby's responsiveness following the birth.

Meanwhile, your baby is busy processing this new experience. Your own instincts will guide you in how best to respond to your baby's initial searching movements. Although a newborn may seem to have little ability to control her muscles, she is capable of a surprising number of responses. Newborns will search out and prefer a face to other objects. She can smell and taste, and quickly learn to distinguish and prefer her mother's breast milk to the milk of other mothers. Reflex movements allow her to reach out for a nipple with her mouth and close her fist over objects to cling and pull herself along. Your own baby may begin to search for the nipple right away and even try to pull it into her mouth. Many babies have been busy sucking their thumbs for months in the womb and they know all about this form of oral satisfaction. Other babies are distracted by the new stimulation of lights and touch. Most babies have a quiet and open expression during the first hour after birth. They seem to be processing the experience their senses provide, feeling the touch of fabrics, skin, and the air around them. Hold your baby and stroke her skin. Her sucking will stimulate hormones that cause uterine contractions that help expel the placenta and stop uterine bleeding, but so will the emotions engendered by this first contact.

Delay as many other procedures as possible during the first hour with your baby. This is the time to enjoy the wonder of new life and the joy you experience in finally seeing and cherishing your baby. Only a few other things must be accomplished before you can completely relax with your baby. While mom is engaged with the third stage of labor and delivering the placenta, dad can continue the bonding process. Great emphasis is placed on the imprinting and bonding that occurs between parents and babies at birth. This moment is special to the new family, but the busy scene in the birth room may require attention to other issues, especially if your baby is born in the hospital. Don't worry. You will have ample opportunity to bond with your baby, even if you must be separated because of health problems or medical procedures. Babies are extremely resilient, and the deep bonds of attachment will develop regardless of what happens at the birth.

Newborn Exams and Procedures

Whether your baby is born at home with a midwife, at a birthing center, or in the hospital, a newborn exam is essential within minutes after birth to establish that vital systems are functioning normally. Someone should listen to the heart and lungs, and inspect the baby's skin, eyes, mouth, spine, and genitalia for congenital problems. This exam can be performed quietly and gently, with the baby cradled in the mother's arms. If mom is busy with other tasks, such as pushing out the placenta, then the father or birth partner can hold the baby. Babies should not be whisked away for measurements.

A medical provider will perform a more detailed physical exam within a few hours of birth. A pediatrician in the hospital or a midwife at home usually fulfills this task. In the hospital, the medical staff may insist that this exam be done in the nursery, but there is no reason why it cannot occur in the mother's room. Do not allow your baby out of your sight. Once your baby is out of your arms, you lose control. Even previous agreements with your doctor can easily go by the wayside when hospital routines begin. Of course, if some form of treatment is required, parents should not interfere, though they should be informed at each step. Most procedures can be easily accomplished with the baby in a parent's arms.

When babies are born at home, the midwife will review each procedure with parents in an informative discussion that provides them with choices. In the hospital, most parents assume that the pediatric staff will do exactly what is needed to ensure their baby's welfare. However, like many other child health issues, a conscious choice may be healthier and safer for your bundle of joy than trusting in the wisdom of medical recommendations. Soon after every baby's birth, a number of hospital procedures are performed on the newborn by the medical staff. If parents are prepared to deal with the typical hospital routines, they can make informed decisions, determining which procedures are appropriate for them and which may be unnecessary. If expectant parents plan ahead, then their baby's first day in the world will reflect their own wishes and judgments. Parents who have considered their options will be at an advantage at the time of their blessed event.

Hospital protocols are written to streamline and standardize patient procedures. They are not individualized to your needs, or intended to create a loving environment that fosters parent-infant bonding. This is not the time for intrusions or invasive procedures. Medical interventions should be kept to a minimum. Birth is a time for family bonding.

If the medical team observes or anticipates problems, then some medical procedures may be necessary. Resuscitation is an emergency procedure that must take precedence over everything else. For an uncomplicated birth, simple suctioning of the airways with a bulb syringe and wiping the baby's eyes are all the interventions necessary before the infant is put into the mother's arms and taken to the breast.

Washing the Newborn

Your baby does not need washing. Most babies are born with a protective layer of vernix covering the skin. This lanolin-like substance is a natural, fatty moisturizer that parents can massage into the skin. Soap washes this protective layer away. Blood and mucus on the baby causes no harm. Your baby should be kept warm next to mom's body, with the head covered to prevent heat loss. A bath is not appropriate. Save the first bath for later when your baby is adjusted to the environment. Protect your baby's eyes from harsh lights and maintain physical contact with your baby's body. The newborn has just emerged from nine months in a dark, aquatic existence, with muffled sounds and close-fitting walls. Allow your baby to adjust slowly and quietly to the world of air, light, and sound.

Eye Medications

The first drugs a baby usually encounters are antibiotic drops or ointment placed in the eyes to prevent sexually transmitted diseases (STDs). Babies sometimes contract gonorrhea or chlamydia when passing through the vaginal canal. Application of antibiotic ointment to an infant's eyes will help prevent transmission of gonorrhea, but will not prevent chlamydia. However, if a mother knows that she is not infected with these STDs (because testing is done for these types of diseases during pregnancy), her baby does not need the drug. The medications themselves can temporarily blur vision and cause eye irritation from toxic reactions, so it is better to avoid them whenever possible. If you wish to refuse these drugs, you may need to sign a waiver in the hospital.

Vitamin K

An injection of vitamin K (1 mg) is routinely administered to all newborns to prevent unexpected bleeding caused by low levels of vitamin K-dependent blood clotting factors. Vitamin K is present in green vegetables, vegetable oils, and dairy products, but intake or supplementation during pregnancy does not ensure prevention of vitamin K deficiency in newborns.

The syndrome of vitamin K deficiency bleeding (VKDB) occurs in approximately one in 10,000 babies. VKDB is typically separated into three categories (early, classic, and late) depending on the age of the infant at onset. Early bleeding, within the first twenty-four hours after birth, cannot be prevented by administration of vitamin K. Classic hemorrhagic disease begins on days one to seven, and bleeding usually occurs in the gastrointestinal tract, the skin, the nose, or from a circumcision. Vitamin K, given by injection or orally, improves blood coagulation, and both methods of administration are presumed to be effective in the prevention of this type of bleeding. Late hemorrhagic disease occurs from week two through twelve. Half of these affected babies suffer sudden bleeding into the brain, and 20 percent of affected babies die. Studies have shown that a single injection or oral dose of vitamin K at birth results in adequate coagulation status and vitamin K levels for up to three months following birth. Interestingly, clinical studies have found that infants given three, weekly oral doses of vitamin K (1 mg) have higher vitamin K levels at two weeks and two months compared to infants given a single vitamin K injection at birth, though their coagulation status showed no differences.

Oral administration of vitamin K is as effective as an injection in maintaining adequate levels of vitamin K in the baby's bloodstream and in maintaining adequate coagulation status. It is assumed that maintenance of these blood levels will prevent bleeding, though complete clinical studies to determine effectiveness have not been accomplished because studies in a disease this rare are prohibitively expensive.

Injected vitamin K ran into a problem when researchers in 1990 noted an increased incidence of childhood cancer in children given vitamin K injections at birth. Specifically, they found that injected vitamin K doubled the incidence of leukemia in children younger than age 10. A subsequent study in 1992 revealed the same association between injected vitamin K and cancer, but no such association with oral vitamin K. These researchers recommended exclusive use of oral vitamin K.

Since vitamin K given within twelve hours of birth can reduce the risk of vitamin K deficiency bleeding, it seems prudent to give an oral dose of 1–2 mg. Injections of vitamin K are painful and can cause bruising at the injection site. There may also be an increased risk of cancer associated with vitamin K injections.

Mothers should eat foods with high vitamin K content during pregnancy (green vegetables, vegetable oils, and dairy products) because vitamin K is transferred to the fetus across the placenta. Pregnant women can also take alfalfa tablets, a good source of vitamin K. This will assure an extra margin of safety in addition to providing vitamin K for your baby after the birth.

It is also advisable to give 1–2 mg of vitamin K to breastfed infants at ages one to two weeks and at four weeks. Formulas are already supplemented with vitamin K. Alternatively, nursing mothers can take a daily dose of vitamin K during the first three months following birth. If nursing mothers take a daily 5-mg vitamin K supplement, their babies' vitamin K status improves through the first twelve weeks of life.

Although oral vitamin K is not licensed for use as a drug by the FDA, drops for oral administration are available. Typically, one drop contains 2 mg of vitamin K. Contact a midwife in your area or a birthing supply company (such as www.birthwithlove.com). Or ask your health care provider to order liquid vitamin K directly from Scientific Botanicals (206-527-5521).

Hepatitis B Vaccination

The hepatitis B vaccine is routinely given to all infants soon after birth, to prevent the spread of hepatitis from mother to infant during the birthing process. Hepatitis B is a viral infection usually acquired during adolescence or adulthood as a result of sexual contact, injection drug use, or occupational or household exposure. Infants born to hepatitis B infected mothers are at high risk of contracting hepatitis. The risk of an infant acquiring hepatitis depends on the mother's hepatitis B antigen status. Infants who become infected at birth have a 90 percent risk of chronic infection, and up to 25 percent will die of chronic liver disease as adults. Children do not commonly contract hepatitis except through family exposure.

Screening pregnant women for HBsAg (hepatitis B surface antigen) will identify those infants at risk of acquiring hepatitis. If a mother is HBsAg negative, then it is extremely unlikely that her child will contract hepatitis B. If a mother tests positive for hepatitis antigen, then parents may choose to give hepatitis vaccine soon after birth, accompanied by hepatitis immune globulin, which provides the infant with active antibodies that begin fighting the virus immediately. Infants born to mothers who are hepatitis-free do not need protection. Parents can refuse the vaccine based on their personal or religious beliefs, even in states where the vaccine is required by law.

The hepatitis B vaccine has been associated with many types of adverse reactions, including diabetes, arthritis, hair loss, bleeding disorders, multiple sclerosis, and death. It is advisable to avoid exposing the newborn's delicate immune and nervous systems to these risks unless the baby's mother has hepatitis.

PKU and Other Blood Tests

All states offer low-cost screening tests for a number of diseases that may be present at birth, and that can cause dangerous symptoms, developmental delays, or death if left untreated. Every state provides testing for all newborns for hypothyroidism and phenylketonuria (PKU). Most states also provide testing for galactosemia and sickle cell disease. Selected states also test for several other congenital diseases.

The tests require a blood sample, usually obtained from a heel prick during the first few days of life, preferably two days or more following birth since tests done too soon can miss some of the diseases. The heel is warmed to increase blood flow and then a small lancet pierces the skin. The blood sample is usually taken on blotter paper, which is then evaluated at a clinical laboratory.

Several of these diseases can be treated by an alteration in diet; others by drugs. The treatment will prevent the complications of the illness, and children will develop normally. Because the tests are relatively noninvasive and because potentially life-threatening illnesses can be discovered and prevented, it is advisable that all infants undergo testing. Even though the diseases themselves are relatively rare, the potential to prevent them warrants this simple procedure.

PKU (phenylketonuria) is caused by congenital absence of the enzyme that breaks down the amino acid phenylalanine. When this amino acid is consumed in the diet, it accumulates in the brain and causes mental retardation and seizures. Normal infant development will occur in these babies if the amino acid is eliminated from the breastfeeding mother's diet and then the child's diet, once solids or formula are introduced. Treatment must be started during the first few days of life to prevent mental retardation. The disease occurs in one of 16,000 babies.

Hypothyroidism can also be detected during the first days of life. Affected infants who receive thyroid hormone treatment will avoid the symptoms of mental retardation caused by the deficiency. The disease occurs in approximately one of 4,000 babies.

Galactosemia is a genetically acquired trait that prevents the infant from metabolizing galactose and lactose, which are present in milk. A strict diet eliminating these sugars will prevent mental retardation. The disease occurs in one of 80,000 babies.

Sickle cell disease is a genetic abnormality resulting in a distorted shape of red blood cells. These inflexible red cells block blood vessels and cause joint pain, abdominal pain, and infections. The disease is most prevalent in black people, where the incidence can be up to one in 375 babies, but sickle cell also occurs in other ethnic groups (particularly Hispanics, Native Americans, and East Indians).

Other screening tests may be appropriate for individuals based on family history and the advice of your health care providers.

Glucose Testing

Hypoglycemia in the newborn (a blood glucose level less than 40 mg/dL) can result in brain damage. Treatment consists of an infusion of glucose delivered by IV. Some babies have a higher risk of developing hypoglycemia than others. Common occurrences of low blood sugar include infants born to diabetic mothers, infants who are small for gestational age, and those who have experienced lack of oxygen during the birth process. Infants in these high-risk categories should be tested for blood glucose levels. Similarly, infants with symptoms suggestive of hypoglycemia such as listlessness, poor muscle tone, or increased heart rate may require testing.

Routine screening of newborns for glucose levels is not recommended because the commonly used screening instruments (Dextrostix and Chemstrips) are unreliable compared to true blood glucose levels. Also, your baby's blood sugar level may be low soon after the birth, but then stabilizes. If low blood sugar does not produce symptoms, then babies do not require treatment for it.

ROUTINE PROCEDURES AND TESTS FOR NEWBORNS

PROCEDURE	RECOMMENDATION
Washing	Not needed
Eye medications	Not needed, unless mother has STD
Vitamin K	Oral 1–2 mg at birth, two weeks, and four weeks
Hepatitis B vaccine	Not recommended, unless mother has hepatitis
PKU and other tests	Yes
Glucose testing	Not recommended, unless in high-risk category

How to Handle Exams and Procedures

Create a checklist of newborn procedures to review with your baby's doctor (see the box). Keep that list handy at the birth. You'll need it. The father or birth partner will take charge of the baby, protect her, and interact with the hospital staff. Just because you have told the pediatrician about your choices does not mean that the hospital staff will comply. They follow strict protocols and routines: Every baby gets a hepatitis B shot and a vitamin K shot. Keep your baby in your arms. Sign the necessary waiver forms. Do not become intimidated by medical providers or allow them to do anything that conflicts with your wishes. Your baby is your responsibility now.

The First Day

It is time for you and your baby to discover each other. What better way than to keep your baby near you, cuddled in your arms? Babies born at home are in the perfect setting, sleeping in their mother's arms. For mothers in the hospital, it takes more planning. Request rooming-in. Your baby needs to be near your body, with easy access to the breast and the comforting presence of her new and permanent caregivers. Your baby has left the aquatic world of a constantly surging maternal heartbeat, muffled sounds of the external world, and a dim orange glow. You can control the transition to a world of bright lights, clear voices, and the touch of fabrics and skin. This is not the time to leave your baby in the hands of strangers, however well meaning and knowledgeable. Your baby needs to discover that you will assist her in the transition to this new world.

Newborns may be alert and observant, staring in apparent wonder at faces, lights, or into empty space. Other babies are overstimulated by so much input and they do little besides sleep. The average newborn sleeps twenty hours each day, which leaves little time for waking interaction with parents. All the more reason to keep your sleeping baby near you. Your baby is learning each moment how to breathe, digest food, and process all the input of the world. Enjoy your first day with your baby by taking a well-deserved rest together. All of you have been through a tumultuous time of labor, birthing, and recovery. Keep your baby with you in bed. She will learn to regulate her breathing and her nursing patterns from your body and your responses to her needs. You will learn her patterns of sleep and waking, and her expressions of hunger or discomfort. Then you can respond to her immediately, establishing the relationship that will continue throughout her infancy.

How long should you stay in the hospital? This will depend on how you feel. Many mothers want to get home to their own familiar nest as soon as possible. Once your baby is stabilized and uterine bleeding has slowed down, there is no medical reason to stay. Often, within a few hours you can be discharged and return home. If you stay overnight in a private room, then you will have a quiet place to attend to your baby.

Some mothers welcome the respite and the pampering that the hospital provides. If you have older children at home, then you may want to consider remaining in the hospital to get acquainted with this new baby before bringing her home and interacting with the family. This would allow your baby some quiet time alone with you to build the nursing relationship free of other distractions. Someone besides dad needs to be available for your other children if mom remains in the hospital for an extended time. Of course, if mom had a cesarean or other complications, then she will need to stay in the hospital for her recovery.

Getting Started with Breastfeeding

Offering the Breast

Offer your breast at the first opportunity. Your baby will come to associate breastfeeding with comfort, love, attention, and the assurance that all is right with the world. When you first hold your baby, place her next to your skin. Let her feel the warmth of your breast on her face. She may lick your breast, nuzzle the nipple, or even open her mouth for a feeding. Her instinctual reflexes guarantee that she will find the breast and know what to do. Your newborn should be free to move her arms and legs, not swaddled tightly in a blanket. This is a time for her to explore and discover.

Here is the best method to begin breastfeeding. Establish this routine and it will become second nature to you and your baby. If you are sitting up, place a pillow beneath your baby so that she is resting at an even level with your breast. If you are lying on your side, you and your baby should be facing each other. Hold your baby in one arm and grasp your breast with the opposite hand, the fingers and thumb causing the areola to puff out. Position your baby's body facing your body. Align her head straight with her spine, not rotated to the side, and not tilted back on her neck. Then allow her to explore your breast with her mouth. She may open her mouth or turn her head, showing that she is ready to nurse. If she does not, then gently rub her lips or her cheek with your finger or nipple. She will turn toward the stimulation or move her head from side to side hunting for her food. You may want to express a few drops of colostrum onto your nipple or her lips so she knows it is there.

The next step is getting her to open her mouth wide. When she does this, you have one second to pull her into the breast. Do not move forward toward her. Bring her quickly toward the breast. Then she will latch on properly with your areola in her mouth. If you miss this opportunity, her mouth will close again. Don't worry. She will give you a second try. Your goal is to get as much of your breast as possible into her mouth while it is wide open. Don't put your nipple in there until she has her mouth open wide. You do not want her chewing or nibbling on the end of your nipple, ever. She will not get a good hold to nurse, and your nipple will get sore. Your baby's tongue will press up against the areola and the milk ducts when she sucks. The resulting suction and pressure on the ducts will cause the milk to flow down into your baby's mouth. If she does not have most of the areola in her mouth, then place a finger between your nipple and her lips to break the suction and begin again. If she brings a hand up between the breast and her mouth, take it away with your cradling hand.

Breastfeeding involves three simple steps:

Position your baby properly, with her body facing yours and her head aligned with her spine.

When her mouth opens, pull her right up to your breast.

Make sure most of the areola is in her mouth—not just the nipple. If not, break the suction, and pull her toward the breast again when her mouth reopens.

Once your baby latches on properly, she will begin to suck. After a few minutes you may feel a tingling sensation in your breast, and the opposite side may begin to leak. These are signs of milk ejection. If you don't feel it, don't worry. Your baby will get all she needs anyway. The first few days of nursing stimulates the production of milk. Immediately after the birth and for the next several days, your breasts produce colostrum, one of nature's most miraculous inventions.

Colostrum

The first substance your baby receives in her newfound world is colostrum. You may have already seen this clear or yellowish thick fluid leaking from your nipple, or expressed it yourself during pregnancy. Colostrum is the greatest immune enhancing substance your baby will ever receive. During pregnancy your antibodies pass from your bloodstream directly to your baby's blood. These antibodies protect your baby for several months from specific microorganisms you have encountered throughout your life. Colostrum also transmits antibodies and other immune enhancing substances to your baby. Even if you are not planning to continue breastfeeding your baby, it is wise to allow her to get your colostrum. During the first few hours after birth, your colostrum contains the highest concentration of immune factors, so this is the ideal time to begin nursing.

What is so special about colostrum? Why is it so essential for your baby? Colostrum contains immune defense factors that actively prevent infections and stimulate your baby's own immune system. The most prominent of these factors is an immunoglobulin, IgA, which resides on mucous membranes such as the intestinal lining and protects the body from invading microorganisms. The concentration of immunoglobulins is highest during the first few hours after birth. White blood cells, leucocytes, are living cells that respond to infection by ingesting bacte-

---

IMMUNE AGENTS CONTAINED IN COLOSTRUM

IgA Immunoglobulins; protect the body from invading organisms

Leucocytes Ingest bacteria and release IgA

Lactoferrin Prevents bacteria from using iron

Lysozyme Destroys bacteria and viruses on contact

Cytokines Stimulate immunoglobulins and T cells

Saccharides Bind to bacteria and prevent infection

---

ria and releasing IgA. Colostrum and breast milk contain as many white cells as the bloodstream. Lactoferrin, an iron binding protein found in colostrum, also protects the body from infection by locking onto iron and releasing the iron to red blood cells, thus preventing bacteria from using the iron required for their reproduction. Lysozyme is an agent found in bodily secretions such as saliva that destroys microorganisms on contact. Its presence in colostrum and breast milk has led infant formula manufacturers to add lysozyme to all formulas. Cytokines regulate the intensity and duration of immune responses, boosting activity of T cells and stimulating production of immunoglobulins. Specific sugars, including oligopolysaccharides and glycoconjugates, bind to bacteria that typically cause ear infections, lung infections, and diarrhea, and block their attachment to mucous membranes. These and other powerful immune factors protect your baby during the critical period of exposure to pathogens in the newborn's first days of life.

Does Your Newborn Need Additional Water or Formula?

It is unwise to give your baby a supplement of formula or water in the newborn period. The primary reason is nipple confusion. You want your baby to learn how to nurse on your breast. Nursing from a plastic nipple involves a different muscle coordination system. Plastic nipples deliver milk with less effort on the baby's part, less tongue action, and less sucking. When confronted again with your breast, she will have difficulty adapting to this form of sucking and become confused about what is required to get milk. Second, if your baby receives bottles, she will nurse less and get less colostrum and its beneficial immune factors. Third, if she nurses less, then it will be more difficult and take longer to develop your milk supply because your breasts increase their production of milk in response to nursing. The more sucking, the more milk. Finally, even one supplemental bottle of formula will begin to change the delicate balance of intestinal bacteria in your baby's immature digestive tract. Inform the hospital staff that you do not want your baby to receive any supplemental bottles—nothing except breast milk.

The Circumcision Decision
Myths and Misconceptions

Surgical circumcision involves the removal of the foreskin of the penis. Routine circumcision is an arcane practice that gained popularity in the Victorian era to reduce the incidence of masturbation in boys. Although the success of the procedure for this purpose was never proven, the sexual importance of the foreskin lends credence to the theory. The foreskin is a source of sexual stimulation. In the past, under the influence of strict moral codes, sexual pleasure was discouraged. Modern views, however, tend to encourage rather than discourage sex and masturbation as beneficial activities rather than harmful or shameful sins. Forms of female genital mutilation similar to male circumcision are prohibited by law. These have included surgical removal of the clitoris and chemical mutilation for a similar purpose, reducing female sexual desire and pleasure.

The other common misperception is that circumcision will assist in cleanliness of the penis and reduce problems associated with poor hygiene, specifically an unpleasant odor and irritation. This may have been a problem in an era or geographical location where water was scarce, but adequate bathing will prevent these symptoms. Ironically, the foreskin serves the useful function of maintaining cleanliness of the head of the penis, not collecting secretions, an argument that is often used to continue the practice of its surgical removal.

The medical profession has sought justification for routine circumcision by attempting to associate various diseases with the uncircumcised penis. Various older studies suggested that circumcision might reduce the incidence of cancer of the penis, cancer of the cervix in women, urinary infections in infants, and sexually transmitted diseases. Modern studies have discounted or disproved the relationship of any of these disease conditions with circumcision. Penile cancer occurs in both circumcised and uncircumcised men. Cervical cancer is associated with hygiene, STDs, and a history of multiple sexual partners—not the foreskin of those sexual partners. Urinary infections are not more common in uncircumcised babies. There is no medical justification for routine circumcision. The American Academy of Pediatrics has concluded that data regarding benefits "are not sufficient to recommend routine neonatal circumcision."

Like any other surgical procedure, circumcision is associated with a number of side effects. The most dangerous side effect is hemorrhage. The discovery by parents of a diaper full of blood is horrifying. This can occur if one of the blood vessels severed during the surgery continues to bleed or opens later at the site of the wound during the inflammatory response that follows surgery. Other common side effects include infection, and inadvertent cuts to the glans or shaft of the penis with subsequent scarring or permanent skin tags.

Function of the Foreskin

The foreskin has two major functions: It protects the head of the penis, and it plays a considerable role in sexual stimulation and intercourse. The foreskin provides protection from urinary tract infections because it covers the glans (head) of the penis and the opening of the urethra. This prevents feces and ammonia in your baby's diaper from irritating the sensitive mucous membranes of the glans and the urethra. Removing the foreskin allows pathogens easier access to the urethra. In addition, the foreskin contains specialized glands that secrete a lubricating fluid to keep the glans moist. This is important because the surface of the glans is similar to that of the gums and eyeball, both of which require protection in order to maintain a moist state. The foreskin is similar to the eyelid in its ability to slide across the glans with its innermost layer and protect the glans with its outer layer of skin. When the foreskin is removed, the glans loses its sensitivity, becoming tough and relatively insensitive.

The foreskin maintains the sexual sensitivity of the glans, but it also provides nerve endings itself—an estimated 20,000 of them. More important, the gliding motion of the foreskin over the shaft of the penis and the glans can produce stimulation. This rolling and gliding mechanism stimulates specialized receptors on the surface of the foreskin during both masturbation and intercourse. The gliding foreskin also contributes to sexual pleasure in the woman and protects the sensitive vaginal membranes from friction and chafing when the foreskin slides over the glans.

The Surgical Procedure

Removal of the foreskin requires that the baby be restrained. A special board is employed to strap the infant down so that he cannot escape or flail during the painful procedure. A general anesthetic cannot be used because it may cause respiratory arrest in infants. Instead a cream containing the analgesics lidocaine and prilocaine is applied to the penis, or a local anesthetic is injected directly into the penis. These endeavors to relieve pain seem to be partially successful. However, studies have shown that crying and elevation of heart rate, two typical reactions to pain, are only diminished by approximately 50 percent. In many ritual religious circumcisions, no anesthetic is used to numb the excruciating pain.

Circumcision is a four-step procedure. First, a blunt probe is used to forcibly separate the foreskin from the underlying glans. This is necessary because at birth the foreskin adheres to the glans. Normally the foreskin will gradually separate from the glans over the first few years of life, allowing complete retraction of the foreskin by the time a boy is about 5 years old. The second step involves cutting the foreskin longitudinally from its tip to the ridge of the glans with a knife or scissors. A clamp or bell structure is then placed over the glans and a tight band or string crushes the foreskin around its circumference. Finally, the foreskin is draped over the bell and cut off with a knife. During the ensuing days, the penis is red, swollen, and painful.

Parental Reasons for Circumcision

Parents are sometimes concerned that leaving the baby intact will require inordinate care and hygiene of the penis. This is not the case since no special care whatsoever is required for the intact penis. No forceful retraction of the foreskin, no special cleaning, no handling at all.

Other parents worry that their son's penis will not look like his father's or his peers'. If parents explain to their son that a painful and disfiguring operation was performed on the father and they have spared their son this operation, and that the foreskin is a useful part of the body, then the boy should be satisfied, and probably grateful. Since nearly 50 percent of American males are not circumcised, it is unlikely that a boy will feel abnormal if his penis is left intact. In most parts of world circumcision is discouraged.

Jewish or Muslim parents may be subject to religious laws that dictate circumcision for all males. Although some religious leaders have questioned the continuation of the ritual, many parents feel compelled by custom, tradition, and strict religious codes that demand circumcision. On the other hand, a growing number of Jewish and Muslim parents now question the validity and appropriateness of circumcision, choosing alternative and more humane forms of ritual to bring their children into the religious covenant.

Care of the Circumcised Penis

When a baby has been circumcised, it is important to be vigilant about bleeding and signs of infection, which include inordinate swelling and the formation of a pussy discharge. Infection can usually be prevented by liberal use of Calendula ointment applied to the diaper where it comes into contact with the penis. Calendula encourages healing of wounds and acts as a natural antiseptic. Give the baby *Arnica* 30c (a homeopathic medicine), two pellets twice a day orally for three days following circumcision, to prevent swelling and promote a healing reaction in the injured tissues.

Prepare for Your Newborn

Prepare for your baby's first day of life. Decide before the birth what you want, and discuss your choices with your birth attendant and your pediatrician or family doctor. Keep your checklist with the birth kit and

NEWBORN CHECKLIST		
	YES	NO
Washing	____	____
Eye medications	____	____
Vitamin K	____	____
Hepatitis B vaccine	____	____
PKU testing	____	____
Glucose testing	____	____
Breastfeeding & breast milk only	____	____
Circumcision	____	____
Rooming-in	____	____

bring it to the hospital. Show it to the nursing staff. Sign waiver forms if necessary for procedures that you choose to decline.

Be prepared and you will avoid confrontations and disappointment. This will enable you to focus on the emotional and spiritual levels of your birthing experience, the joy, the amazement, and the love.

CHAPTER 6

Your New Baby

What You Will Need

By now you have been amassing baby paraphernalia, but the list of essential items is short. You will need a few receiving blankets to swaddle your baby, a few knit caps to keep his head warm, a good supply of cotton shirts and onesies, cloth diapers with covers, a pack of nontoxic diaper wipes, a car seat, and a sling. That's about it. Buy all-cotton clothes. You can even find everything in organic cotton. Approximately one pound of pesticides is used on the cotton to make a single T-shirt. Good sources for organic and environmentally friendly products are www.hpakids.org, www.mothering.com, and the book *Guide to Natural Baby Care*, by Mothers and Others for a Livable Planet. Or you can simply do an Internet search on organic baby clothes and find everything you need. Synthetic fabrics are treated with the volatile organic compounds (VOCs) formaldehyde, benzene, and toluene, which come in contact with your baby's sensitive skin and emit gases your baby will breathe. Beware of baby sleepwear, which must be treated for fire safety. Sleepwear comes in two varieties: It is either made of synthetic fibers designed to be flame-resistant or made of cotton and designed to fit snugly so that it is less likely to contact flames or allow an air space for oxygen between the fabric and skin.

Shopping Lists

BABY CLOTHES:

10 cotton shirts

4 cotton onesies with crotch snaps

6 pairs of booties and socks

3 cotton knit caps

SUPPLIES:

Car seat

Diapers

12 diaper covers

Nontoxic baby wipes

6 cotton receiving blankets

Sling

Baby bathtub

Nontoxic shampoo, soaps, and lotions

Chlorine bath ball

You can collect lots of baby stuff, and your relatives will continue to send baby clothes and hand-me-downs. Accept them with good cheer. Buy the baby things you will need for the first few weeks and then see how you feel about outfitting him for the rest of his life.

There are many items you don't need. You don't need a baby bed. You don't need a changing table. You don't even need a separate room for your baby, though of course you will want one eventually.

Don't forget to use nontoxic paints when preparing the baby's room. You might need some drawers in a dresser for baby clothes. A plastic baby bath, with a chlorine removal ball for clean water, is a good idea. A bottle of organic, environmentally friendly baby shampoo and organic lotions or creams are a nice touch.

Your newborn baby needs lots of love, attention, breast milk, and holding. Mothers need to rest and drink lots of fluids during the postpartum period. Arrange for family and friends to take care of the new mom for a few weeks. If dad can stay at home with the nursing couple, all the better. Wear your baby during the day and for outings. Sleep with your newborn in the bed and take naps with your baby. Mothers need to be replenished after the work of pregnancy and birthing. Plenty of rest and good nutrition will restore mothers to their peak of energy. Chinese medicine offers time-honored herbal formulas for restoring chi and blood. Consult your own natural medicine provider about a plan to maintain good health during the postpartum and nursing phase of your life.

Diapers: Cloth or Disposable?

Your newborn will use 10–15 diapers per day, not including the diapers used for spitting up and breast milk overflow. I recommend cloth diapers for newborns because of the sheer volume. Your newborn will pee every time he breastfeeds. Support your local diaper service if you have one in your area. You can find one in the yellow pages or through www.diapernet.com, the website of the National Association of Diaper Services. Order diapers prior to baby's birth and they will be there ready for you when your baby is born. Even if you don't have a diaper service in your area, consider using cotton diapers and washing your own. You will need 3–5 dozen cloth diapers. You will also need a supply of diaper covers (10–12), whether you have diaper service or wash your own. These come in wool or cotton wraparounds that close in front with Velcro or snaps. Cotton covers come with a polyester moisture shield. Thick wool covers are naturally waterproof. Try different styles and see which you prefer. Search for "natural diaper covers" on the Internet for suppliers.

Once your baby is older and using fewer diapers, you may want to switch to disposables. Keep in mind that 18 *billion* diapers are deposited in landfills every year, according to the EPA. This landfill includes untreated human waste. Diaper service and disposable diapers will cost you about the same amount, but the burden to the environment of disposables is considerable. Another option is to use cloth diapers during the day and disposable diapers at night, when you want more absorbency. Some parents object to the idea of putting the chemicals contained in disposable diapers next to their baby's skin. Disposable diapers contain chlorine, which contributes to dioxins in the environment, and polymer gel granules to absorb water. Tushies makes a chlorine-free, polymer-free diaper composed of cotton and wood pulp. Seventh Generation also has a chlorine-free diaper.

The First Weeks

You will be busy the first week at home with your baby, enjoying this new addition to the family, adjusting to a completely different routine, recovering yourself, feeding him, and making sure that all systems are working normally. That's a lot to do. Get all the help you can, and limit visitors as much as possible. This is the time for you to get your equilibrium and focus on your baby. You will have plenty of time to show your baby to legions of friends and relatives. Now you need to rest and cuddle with your newborn. Mothers in this recovery period should not be cooking, cleaning, doing laundry, or caring for the older children.

Your baby needs your full attention and your body needs to recover from the fluid and energy drain of birth and nursing. This is your time to regain your strength. You will need it. Sleep with your baby during the day. He will be waking you often in the night to nurse. Do not leave your baby alone to sleep. He needs to be next to your body.

Keep your baby's head covered with a knitted cap. Babies lose most of their body heat through their heads and newborns may not always have good temperature control. A baby that weighs 8 pounds or more usually has adequate temperature regulation. In colder weather, always put a cap on your baby when outdoors.

Your baby will begin passing meconium within the first day after birth. This is a sticky, dark green, tar-like substance. The stools will gradually change from green to brown to yellow over the next few days. Your baby should be having regular bowel movements—usually several a day, sometimes more. The consistency of a breastfed baby's stool is pasty to watery, bright yellow to mustardy in color, often with white seedy curds of milk. Green stools are not unusual in babies. And sometimes a baby will decide to go a few days without any stools. All of these variations are normal. Just make sure your baby does pass stools. If he has not had a bowel movement by the second day after birth, contact your medical provider. Your baby will usually pee every time he nurses. If you use paper diapers, they may not seem wet because of the diaper's absorbency, but they should be changed nonetheless. Leaving wet diapers in contact with your baby's skin tends to cause diaper rash.

Your baby may be born with peeling skin, or his skin may start to peel soon after birth. Some babies start off with acne—red bumps or white bumps, sometimes a few, sometimes a zillion. The only thing you need to do for your baby's skin is to wash in the folds and cracks to prevent rashes. Keep your baby's diaper off sometimes in a warm room to let his skin breathe. He will enjoy the freedom. If you see any sign of diaper rash, use a diaper cream made by Weleda, Mustela, or from a similarly nontoxic source.

Begin massaging your baby from an early age. Gently rub the inside and outside of the arms and legs to stimulate the acupuncture channels. This form of massage will encourage normal development of your baby's organ systems, especially digestive functions. Rub his abdomen with the flat of your palm in a counter-clockwise direction to encourage health digestion. Turn your baby over and rub along the sides of his spine from the neck down to the buttocks. Then rub down the backs of his thighs and legs. This downward motion strengthens the bladder channel and will help build your baby's fundamental energetic resources.

Weight Gain

During the first week your baby will lose weight until breastfeeding is well established. Typically, babies lose 6 to 10 ounces, or 5 to 8 percent of their body weight, in the first week. Babies are born with extra fluids and fat to enable this weight loss with no adverse effect on their health. Your baby should be back to his birth weight within two to three weeks. After that, the average baby will gain 6 to 8 ounces per week, or about 2 pounds per month, for the first three months. After six months, your baby will gain about a pound each month. If you are concerned about your baby's weight gain, you can obtain a very accurate weight between medical checkups by putting your baby on the checkout scale at your grocery store. Grocery clerks are usually happy to have the diversion of weighing babies. You can obtain the same growth charts that medical providers use by searching for "growth charts" on the Internet. The weight you obtain with your clothed baby will be greater than his naked weight at the doctor's office. If you have any concerns about your baby's weight gain or your milk supply, contact your medical provider.

Jaundice

Jaundice is a yellow tinge of the skin and eyeballs that often occurs in the first week of a baby's life. The word *jaundice* is derived from the French word *jaune,* or yellow. Most babies become jaundiced and the yellow color gradually fades away. This yellow tinge is caused by a normal process of the breakdown of red blood cells. Babies are born with more red cells than they need, so their body naturally begins breaking down the extra cells. When red cells break down, one of their constituents, bilirubin, is released into the bloodstream. Normally the liver disposes of the excess bilirubin, but a baby's immature liver cannot handle the overload. This excess bilirubin collects in the skin and turns it yellow. Generally, the higher the bilirubin level in the blood, the more deeply yellow or orange the skin will appear, although darkly pigmented infants may not appear significantly jaundiced even though bilirubin levels are high. Extremely high levels of bilirubin can cause brain damage—the primary reason to be concerned about jaundice. If jaundice appears in the first twenty-four hours, it may be caused by a difference in blood types between mother and baby. This incompatibility of blood can result in the mother creating antibodies against the baby's blood type. The antibodies will cause an excessive breakdown of red blood cells. Babies with these blood incompatibilities and those with a few other medical conditions are at higher risk of developing problems.

If your baby appears yellow, your medical provider may choose to perform a blood test to measure bilirubin levels. Based on the level of bilirubin detected and your baby's age in hours, the doctor will decide whether to recommend treatment. Typical treatment consists of light therapy, or phototherapy. The baby's skin is exposed to light generated by lamps. The blue spectrum of the light breaks down the bilirubin in the skin. Ultraviolet light has no effect and is not used. Phototherapy can be administered at home or in a hospital with specially designed fluorescent lights or other bulbs, or through a fiber-optic system contained in a blanket wrapped around the baby. Your baby can also be placed naked in the sunlight streaming through a window. The glass will filter the ultraviolet light that causes sunburn.

It is very important for jaundiced babies to continue breastfeeding. Fluid intake helps babies flush out bilirubin. Do not stop breastfeeding because of jaundice, and do not allow any treatment to interfere with nursing. It is important to build the milk supply during the first week; interrupting the schedule of regular nursing will cause a decline in the milk supply. Babies do not need formula or water because of jaundice.

The homeopathic medicine *Chelidonium* can be safely used to treat jaundice, in addition to phototherapy.

Bathing and Hygiene

Keeping your baby clean sounds easy, but in practice it takes some attention. Babies have sensitive skin that is easily irritated by milk that dribbles into folds of skin or a dirty diaper in contact with the skin for too long. Newborn babies have a protective whitish coating called vernix that is a natural moisturizer. You can massage this vernix into your baby's skin during the first day or two after the birth. Once your baby starts nursing and pooping, you will need to start keeping him clean. Wipe your baby with warm water and a washcloth. Be sure to clean in the folds of skin at his neck, underarms, elbows, groin, and knees. When changing girls' diapers, gently spread the labia and wipe in the crevices from front to back with a moistened cotton ball. If you gently spread apart the inner labia, you will prevent them from fusing together, a development that can cause minor problems and is easily prevented. A boy's penis requires no special treatment. Do not attempt to retract the foreskin at any age.

Sponge baths are appropriate for babies until the cord stump falls off, usually one to two weeks after birth. The cord does not need any special attention. It is best to keep the cord dry. A sponge bath is easily accomplished with a washcloth and a mild soap or shampoo. (See page 73 on choosing baby products for the bath.) Spread a towel, fill a mixing bowl with warm water, and you're all set. You can rinse your baby in the sink, or you can accomplish the entire task in a baby bathtub.

Once your baby is ready for immersion in a bath, you can hold him in your lap in the tub, or hold him in the sink, or lay him in a baby tub. When you take a bath with your baby, be very careful not to slip when taking your baby into or out of the tub. If you use the sink, spread a small towel on the bottom or use a plastic insert or non-slip mat. Some babies love the water, others become anxious. Sooner or later they learn that baths are great fun.

To clean babies after removing a dirty diaper, use water and a cloth or non-alcohol wipes (available at larger health food stores and made by Seventh Generation or Tushies). Here is a suggestion about how to make your own baby wipes, courtesy of Ruth Yaron, from her book *Super Baby Food*. Make a solution of 2 cups water, 2 tablespoons baby shampoo, 1 tablespoon aloe vera gel, and 8 drops lavender oil. Take a stack of white paper towels available at discount stores. Put them in a suitable plastic container. Dump in the solution. If they get dry, add some water. If they are too wet, leave the top off for a while.

Breastfeeding

Breast milk is usually the only food your baby will need for the first six months, and you can continue nursing well beyond that age. I encourage mothers to breastfeed for at least twelve months. However, nursing your toddler will still provide your growing child with the beneficial effects of breast milk. The milk from your breast is the ideal food for your baby. Babies fed anything other than breast milk have dramatically altered intestinal bacteria and lower gut pH. They have a much greater chance of developing allergic reactions and digestive disturbances. This is unfortunately true for babies exclusively fed formula or supplemented with occasional bottles of formula. It takes several months for your baby's intestinal tract to develop the tightly closed junctions of the intestinal mucosal cells that protect the gut from foreign proteins and bacteria. Prior to that time the introduction of cow's milk proteins can trigger irritation and allergic reactions that may persist for years.

Breastfed babies have fewer infections, a lower incidence of allergy and asthma into early childhood (Oddy et al., 2004), less obesity later in life (Gillman et al., 2001), and a higher IQ (Oddy et al., 2003) than formula fed children. This advantage in intelligence persists for breastfed children into their adult years (Mortensen et al., 2002). Breast milk enhances immune function in children, and this immune protection persists for years after breastfeeding is discontinued (Hanson, 1998). Babies fed cow's milk proteins have an increased risk of developing insulin dependent diabetes (Karjalainen et al., 1992; Kostraba et al., 1993).

Breastfeeding mothers need to eat a healthy diet in order to maintain an adequate milk supply and supply the proper nutrients to babies through breast milk. A diet with plenty of fresh fruits and vegetables, dairy products made from whole milk, protein from beans, nuts, and organic animal products (chicken, turkey, beef, and pork), and whole grains should be maintained throughout the breastfeeding period. Fish and shrimp should not be consumed by nursing women (except for sardines and wild Alaskan salmon or organic farmed salmon). To ensure proper brain development in babies, mothers should take an omega-3 fatty acid supplement, either 1 tablespoon of cod liver oil or fish oil capsules equivalent to at least 1,500 mg of EPA and 400 mg DHA per day. Mothers should also eat two organic eggs per day and drink 16 ounces

DAILY SUPPLEMENTS FOR NURSING MOTHERS

1 tablespoon cod liver oil, or fish oil capsules equivalent to 1,500 mg EPA and 400 mg DHA

Two organic eggs

16 ounces whole milk (raw or non-homogenized, organic)

Calcium citrate or lactate, 1,000 mg with magnesium

Prenatal multi-vitamin

of raw milk or non-homogenized, pasteurized whole milk per day. A prenatal supplement derived from quality sources is also advisable, plus 1,000 mg calcium citrate or calcium lactate with magnesium.

Nurse your newborn baby as often as he wants, and at least every two hours. Make sure he latches onto the nipple well, to help prevent sore nipples. Burp him after feeding for fifteen minutes on each breast. Your baby will nurse at his own rate and frequency. Allow him to take the lead. If he is a lazy nurser, he may need some encouragement, but most babies are eager to nurse and ready for action upon waking and whenever they feel hungry. As a first-time mother you may have difficulties establishing a routine and finding your way in the nursing relationship. This is the time to seek counsel from breastfeeding experts. Many books and resources are available for breastfeeding moms, and your personal library should contain some of these books for guidance and reference. You will find a list of these books in the appendix. Your local chapter of La Leche League (www.lalecheleague.org), lactation consultants (www.ilca.org), and breastfeeding websites (www.breastfeeding.com) all exist to support you and your baby while you are nursing.

Do not give your baby water or any other supplemental feeding unless advised to do so by your medical provider and lactation consultant. Babies may sometimes seem hungry even after nursing. This might be due to a number of causes, but it is common for babies to nurse more when they experience a growth spurt. Their increased nursing causes an increase in the milk supply. Mothers often mistake this increase in demand for an insufficient milk supply. They seek to satisfy their baby's hunger by giving supplemental formula and their milk supply decreases as a result of the less frequent nursing. This can lead to more bottles, more dependence on formula, and an early termination of breastfeeding. If you are concerned about the sufficiency of your milk supply, consult a provider who can counsel you about nutrition, herbs, and homeopathic treatment. A number of herbs can help build the milk supply. These include fennel seed (*Foeniculum vulgare*), fenugreek seed (*Trigonella foenum-graecum*), borage leaf (*Borago officinalis*), blessed thistle root (*Cnicus benedictus*), and hops flowers (*Humulus lupus*).

Most herbs are safe to use during breastfeeding, and babies rarely show any adverse reactions to herbs transferred through breast milk. The rare reactions in babies whose mothers have taken herbs are usually caused by contaminants or the mistaken use of toxic plants. Some plants and medicinal herbs do have toxicity and their use should be carefully researched with the help of authoritative books and knowledgeable practitioners. Essential oils can cause problems in infants and should only be used with proper guidance. Beware of older, traditional herbal texts that may contain inaccurate information about herbal use during breastfeeding.

The American Botanical Council, in cooperation with Integrative Medicine Communications, published a comprehensive guide to therapeutic herbs (Blumenthal et al., 1998). Herbs to avoid during your breastfeeding period include:

Aloe

Buckthorn bark

Buckthorn berry

Caraway oil

Cascara Sagrada bark

Coltsfoot leaf

Indian snakeroot

Kava Kava

Peppermint oil

Petasites root

Rhubarb root

Sage

Senna leaf

Uva Ursi

If your new baby does need supplemental feedings, then use a supplemental nursing device with a bag and a tube that sits adjacent to your nipple during nursing (Internet sources include www.lact-aid.com and www.medela.com). This will avoid nipple confusion from bottles, eliminate the need to buy and sterilize bottles, and encourage your baby to suck at your breast to continue building the milk supply. If you express milk for someone else to give to your baby, then you will need to purchase glass bottles with silicone nipples.

You can express milk by hand, with a hand pump or an electric pump. If you are working outside the home and expressing your milk on a regular basis, you will want to have an electric pump with two suction devices so that you can express both breasts simultaneously. Refrigerate or freeze breast milk immediately. A bottle of room-temperature breast milk can be used for up to two hours. A bottle of refrigerated milk can be used for up to five days. A bottle of frozen milk four months. Do not, however, defrost and then refreeze breast milk because bacteria may contaminate the milk. To defrost milk, place the bottle of frozen milk in a bowl of warm water. Do not heat milk on the stove, and never heat breast milk in a microwave oven. Milk should never be heated above body temperature. Babies can drink a bottle of milk straight out of the refrigerator.

If your baby enjoys sucking between nursing sessions, try offering your finger to suck on, nail-side down. Once the nursing relationship is well established, after a few weeks you can also use a pacifier. I recommend a silicone nipple that is flattened to simulate the shape of the breast nipple.

If Formula Is Necessary

There is no question that mothers should breastfeed their babies if at all possible. Even if mothers know they will not be able to continue breastfeeding, babies who are started off in life with breast milk will derive tremendous health benefits. Plan to breastfeed as long as possible. Even partial breastfeeding will confer enormous benefits to your baby. If you must go to work outside the home, you can still express milk and feed your baby stored breast milk. Many mothers manage to work at an outside job and also exclusively feed their babies breast milk. If you also need to supplement your baby with formula, you can still continue to breastfeed when you are at home. Remember that formulas are only crude approximations of breast milk, and even the best of formulas fall far short of the remarkable formulation of mother's milk.

There are a few situations where breastfeeding may be difficult or impossible. Mothers of adopted babies can develop their own supply of breast milk, but lactating without a pregnancy and birth is a difficult and time intensive project. Mothers attempting to nurse an adopted baby will also need a supplemental milk supply. Find a lactation consultant knowledgeable in this field. You will also need a supplemental nursing device that allows your baby to receive milk through a tube placed next to your nipple during nursing (available on the Internet at www.lact-aid.com or www.medela.com). Babies and mothers derive comfort, satisfaction, and emotional benefits from the nursing relationship, even beyond the nutritional aspect of breastfeeding. A supplemental nursing device can be used at any time that the breast milk supply is inadequate for the baby's nutritional needs. This simple device will avoid nipple confusion and enable your baby to continue nursing. Mothers who must take medications that contraindicate breastfeeding will also need a secondary source of milk.

If you need to find a supplemental milk source, the first resource to investigate is a local breast milk bank. La Leche League, your hospital, or medical provider can help you locate a source. A doctor's prescription is necessary to purchase donor milk from a milk bank. Concerns about the spread of diseases through breast milk have made it more difficult to find local breast milk banks, but parents can be assured that safety standards are extremely high at these facilities. In times past, parents could hire a wet nurse.

The only other alternative is formula. You can make your own formula, or you can purchase a commercial formula. I have included the formula recipes developed by Sally Fallon and Mary Enig, nutritionists extraordinaire, with their kind permission. These formulas are reprinted from their book, *Nourishing Traditions*, and can also be found on their website at www.westonaprice.org, in the children's health section.

MILK-BASED FORMULA

MAKES 36 OUNCES

This milk-based formula takes account of the fact that human milk is richer in whey, lactose, vitamin C, niacin, and long-chain polyunsaturated fatty acids compared to cow's milk but leaner in casein (milk protein). The addition of gelatin to cow's milk formula will make it more digestible for the infant. Use only truly expeller-expressed oils in the formula recipes, otherwise they may lack vitamin E.

The ideal milk for baby, if he can't be breastfed, is clean, whole raw milk from old-fashioned cows, certified free of disease, that feed on green pasture. For sources of good quality milk, see www.realmilk.com or contact a local chapter of the Weston A. Price Foundation.

If the only choice available to you is commercial milk, choose whole milk, preferably organic and unhomogenized, and culture it with a piima or kefir culture to restore enzymes (available from G.E.M. Cultures 707-964-2922).

2 cups whole milk, preferably unprocessed milk from pasture-fed cows

1/4 cup homemade liquid whey (see recipe for whey, below)

4 tablespoons lactose*

1 teaspoon bifidobacterium infantis**

2 or more tablespoons good quality cream (not ultrapasteurized), more if you are using milk from Holstein cows

1 teaspoon regular dose cod liver oil or 1/2 teaspoon high-vitamin cod liver oil*

1 teaspoon expeller-expressed sunflower oil*

1 teaspoon extra virgin olive oil*

2 teaspoons coconut oil*

2 teaspoons Frontier brand nutritional yeast flakes*

2 teaspoons gelatin*

1 7/8 cups filtered water

1/4 teaspoon acerola powder*

*Available from Radiant Life 888-593-8333 (4radiantlife.com)

**Available from Natren 800-992-3323 or Radiant Life 888-593-8333

Add gelatin to water and heat gently until gelatin is dissolved. Place all ingredients in a very clean glass or stainless steel container and mix well. To serve, pour 6 to 8 ounces into a very clean glass bottle, attach nipple, and set in a pan of simmering water. Heat until warm but not hot to the touch, shake bottle well, and feed baby. (Never, **never** heat formula in a microwave oven!) Note: If you are using the Lact-Aid, mix all ingredients well in a blender.)

VARIATION: GOAT MILK FORMULA

Although goat milk is rich in fat, it must be used with caution in infant feeding as it lacks folic acid and is low in vitamin B_{12}, both of which are essential to the growth and development of the infant. Inclusion of nutritional yeast to provide folic acid is essential. To compensate for low levels of vitamin B_{12}, if preparing the Milk-Based Formula (above) with goat's milk, add *2 teaspoons frozen organic raw chicken liver, finely grated* to the batch of formula. Be sure to begin egg-yolk feeding at four months.

LIVER-BASED FORMULA

MAKES ABOUT 36 OUNCES

The liver-based formula also mimics the nutrient profile of mother's milk. It is extremely important to include coconut oil in this formula as it is the only ingredient that provides the special medium-chain saturated fats found in mother's milk. As with the milk-based formula, all oils should be truly expeller-expressed.

3 3/4 cups homemade (or commercial organic) beef or chicken broth

2 ounces organic liver, cut into small pieces

5 tablespoons lactose*

1 teaspoon bifidobacterium infantis**

1/4 cup homemade liquid whey (see recipe for whey, below)

1 tablespoon coconut oil*

1 teaspoon cod liver oil or 1/2 teaspoon high-vitamin cod liver oil*

1 teaspoon unrefined sunflower oil*

2 teaspoons extra virgin olive oil

1 teaspoon acerola powder

*Available from Radiant Life 888-593-8333

**Available from Natren 800-992-3323

Simmer liver gently in broth until the meat is cooked through. Liquefy using a handheld blender or in a food processor. When the liver broth has cooled, stir in remaining ingredients. Store in a very clean glass or stainless steel container. To serve, stir formula well and pour 6 to 8 ounces in a very clean glass bottle. Attach a clean nipple and set in a pan of simmering water until formula is warm but not hot to the touch, shake well, and feed to baby. (Never heat formula in a microwave oven!)

FORTIFIED COMMERCIAL FORMULA

MAKES ABOUT 35 OUNCES

This stopgap formula can be used in emergencies, or when the ingredients for home-made formula are unavailable.

1 cup low-iron, milk-based powdered formula

29 ounces filtered water ($3^5/8$ cups)

1 large egg yolk from an organic egg, cooked $3^1/2$ minutes

1 teaspoon cod liver oil or $^1/2$ teaspoon high-vitamin cod liver oil

Place all ingredients in a blender or food processor and blend thoroughly. Place 6–8 ounces in a very clean glass bottle. (Store the rest in a very clean glass jar in the refrigerator for the next feedings.) Attach a clean nipple to the bottle and set in a pan of simmering water until formula is warm but not hot to the touch, shake well, and feed to baby. (Never heat formula in a microwave oven!)

Making your own formula is a commitment equivalent to the time and energy you would invest in breastfeeding, but your baby' health will profit from your efforts.

The next alternative is powdered organic formula. Two companies currently produce an organic milk-based formula, Horizon and Nature's One (www.horizonorganic.com and www.naturesone.com). These formulas are preferable to most commercially available formulas, but they will require supplementation as outlined here.

If your baby reacts badly to milk-based formulas, then you can try the organic liver formula described here or discuss the options of other hypo-allergenic milk formulas available to you (Nutramigen, Alimentum).

HOMEMADE WHEY

ABOUT 5 CUPS

Homemade whey is easy to make from good-quality plain yogurt, or from raw or cultured milk. You will need a large strainer that rests over a bowl.

If you are using yogurt, place 2 quarts in the strainer lined with a tea towel. Cover with a plate and leave at room temperature overnight. The whey will drip out into the bowl. Place the whey in clean glass jars and store in the refrigerator.

If you are using raw or cultured milk, place 2 quarts of the milk in a glass container and leave at room temperature for 2–4 days, until the milk separates into curds and whey. Pour into the strainer lined with a tea towel and cover with a plate. Leave at room temperature overnight. The whey will drip out into the bowl. Store in clean glass jars in the refrigerator.

Never give your baby soy formula under any circumstances (see page 51 for a discussion of soy products).

Use only glass bottles for formula or expressed breast milk. (See page 70 for a discussion of plastic bottles.) Use a silicone (clear) nipple with a flattened shape that mimics your breast nipple.

Digestion

Infants are ruled by their stomachs. Hunger is their motivating force, and the quest for nourishment propels their activities. The rooting reflex ensures that your baby will find the breast. Rub his cheek and his head turns and mouth opens, searching for the fulfillment of nursing. Most of his energy is spent digesting breast milk. The child is centered in the digestive tract. When digestion is proceeding well, your baby is content, alert, inquisitive, and sleeping soundly. If digestive function is upset, your baby's nervous system becomes stressed and you may see symptoms of gas, spitting up, diarrhea, tension, and crying. This condition is usually known as infantile colic. As babies grow, their viral illnesses frequently begin with digestive symptoms—a stomach ache or vomiting.

Reflux and excessive spitting up are symptoms of a more disturbed digestive system. Stomach energy descends. If the stomach is weakened, then the digestive tract will not have the strength to propel energy downward.

The treatment for these conditions employs several principles. First, do things that calm and comfort your baby. Second, avoid things that aggravate the symptoms (especially foods in the mother's diet). And third, give your baby natural medicines and supplements that will strengthen and settle digestive function.

Comforting your baby is accomplished primarily by holding and motion. Your baby has been rocked by your body's motion for nine months. He will feel soothed by the same fluid sensation of being in your arms or a sling while you walk him or gently jostle him at your shoulder. Even conventional studies have shown that holding your baby is an effective treatment for crying. Often putting pressure on a baby's abdomen will help relieve tension there. Hold your baby face down with his body stretched along the length of your arm. Or fold your baby's legs against his tummy while in your arms, either facing toward you or facing outward. Swaddling your baby in a receiving blanket during the first month is an excellent way to make him feel secure, and it actually helps to prevent colic. Newborns like to be wrapped in your arms or in a blanket. When babies are wrapped in a blanket, they tend to wake less often, and swaddling increases the amount of REM sleep (Gerard et al., 2002). They sleep better and cry less. Wrap your baby with his arms across his chest, not down at his sides.

SAMANTHA'S SCREAMING: A CASE HISTORY

Pity the poor infant with disturbed digestion. Not only is she subject to colicky pain, intense crying episodes, and spitting up inordinate amounts of stomach acid that burns the esophagus, but she is pumped with drugs that decrease gas and stop stomach acid secretions. These drugs do nothing to cure the problem—a weak digestive system. If parents are not careful, their baby will end up on formula that aggravates the problem further. Such was the fate of Samantha.

For the first three weeks of her life Samantha was fine. Then all hell broke loose. The main problem was screaming in the evenings. Without fail from 5:00 until 8:00 at night Samantha cried. Not the fussy crying that her parents could relieve by gentle rocking and carrying, but full-out screaming that exhausted everyone. This pattern persisted for the next two months with no end in sight. After breastfeeding Samantha required special handling. If her mother did not keep her upright and perfectly quiet, she would spit up most of her meal. She squirmed and pulled up her legs in pitiable efforts to relieve the pain. This led to a drastic alteration of Mom's diet in an attempt to eliminate possible culprits. Out went the dairy products, beans, broccoli, chocolate, spices, garlic, and onions. No effect. The doctor was alarmed because Samantha was not gaining enough weight. "We have

Babies that are gassy and fussy may be aggravated by something in mom's diet. Everything that mothers eat travels through their breast milk, and foods have many potential irritants that upset babies or cause gas. Try eliminating the most common foods known to aggravate colic: dairy products, beans, broccoli and cabbage, nuts, spices, onions, garlic, chocolate, and caffeine. If your baby improves when you eliminate these foods, then reintroduce one at a time and observe your baby's behavior. The most common culprit is dairy, so that should be the first to eliminate and the last to reintroduce.

to reduce her symptoms so she keeps her food down," she said. Then she prescribed two different stomach acid inhibitors, which had little noticeable effect. When she began talking about changing Samantha to a formula, Mom rebelled.

Samantha's dad did an Internet search for reflux and discovered several articles about successful homeopathic treatment. With nothing to lose and a bit of hope, they located a homeopath in their area and took the plunge. The homeopath determined that, despite Samantha's intense screaming, her problem was really not that severe and could probably be easily cured. He cautioned that treatment would need to continue for the next six months, but they would probably see effects soon. The problem was an immature, weak, and damaged digestive tract. He then prescribed *Lycopodium 200*, a homeopathic medicine often used for these symptoms that would correct the underlying imbalance. A Chinese herbal formula, Grow and Thrive, would support the Spleen/Stomach (digestive) system, relieve accumulation of Dampness, and stimulate the smooth passage of food. A *bifidus* supplement would also ensure an adequate supply of intestinal bacteria.

Over the next two months, Samantha became calmer and less frantic. She kept her feedings down, and everyone started sleeping better and crying less. Samantha's parents were frankly amazed at the change, but their homeopath just smiled.

Other treatments can be found in the colic section on page 225. If you suspect digestive problems, the first thing to introduce is a supplement of *Lactobacillus bifidus,* 1/4 teaspoon dissolved in a little breast milk. Give your baby this solution once a day with an eye dropper. Homeopathic medicines usually work well to relieve symptoms. Start with *Colocynth,* especially if your baby seems better when you press on his abdomen. Other medicines—*Nux vomica, Calcarea,* or *Jalapa*—may also be useful.

CHAPTER 7

Four to Nine Months

This is the age when babies begin establishing emotional relationships. By the end of the third month babies have oriented themselves to the world, and established regular patterns of breastfeeding and sleep. Now they are ready to explore their world, rolling over, reaching for objects, and engaging you in "conversations." A 4-month-old is ready for an emotional relationship. Cooing, oohing, and getting your attention with a focused gaze. This baby means to make contact. Your infant now wants to build a familiar exchange of dialogue. You make a face and she makes a face, you babble in that special baby talk and she gurgles right back at you. This is a relationship made in heaven. Everyone is content, everyone in love. Now your baby is ready to explore the world in perfect confidence that you and she have a secure emotional bond that she can depend on. She cries, you are there. Reassured and trusting, she can get on with the serious jobs of finding her toes, directing her hand to a toy, doing that first push-up, and all the other games that lead to mobility and self-reliance. During this stage your baby begins reaching out for things in the world. She will reach for brightly colored toys, begin to twirl your hair while nursing, and try to take food from you when you eat.

Nutrition and Babies
Introducing Solid Foods

At five to six months it is time to start introducing your baby to the idea that some objects in the world, other than a breast or bottle, taste good. Give your baby tastes of food on your finger or on a small spoon if she expresses any interest. Usually she will make a face and push the food back out at you with her tongue. It takes practice for babies to learn how to swallow solids because a new skill of muscular coordination is necessary to get those solids from the tongue into the throat. Up until now your baby has only ingested food by sucking. There is no urgency to get solid foods into your baby at any particular age. Babies do fine on just breast milk for nine months. Some babies are more interested in solids than others. Some 6-month-olds will be grabbing the food out of your hand, while others seem to show no interest at all. Follow your baby's clues, and keep offering different types of foods. Do not feel compelled to get your baby to eat. Giving too many solids may discourage your baby from the all-important task of breastfeeding.

The first foods for babies, other than breast milk or formula, should be egg yolks, cooked fruits, and mashed bananas. Simple carbohydrates are the easiest foods for your baby to digest. The enzymes that break down solid foods develop slowly. Start with very simple carbohydrates and gradually introduce more complex carbohydrates and proteins later. Do not start your baby with rice cereal. Grains are too complex, and the early introduction of grains is associated with later development of allergies. Go slowly, introducing one new food at a time. Then wait two or three days to observe reactions and introduce another.

Common allergic reactions are a rash around the mouth or anus, runny nose, diarrhea, or fussiness. Allow your baby to play with new foods and observe her face afterwards to see if she develops a rash. The most allergenic foods are egg whites, dairy products, nuts, wheat, soy, corn, citrus, and berries.

Infants should get only pureed or mashed foods. Any foods with chunks can cause choking, which is a very serious danger. Of course you need to be vigilant about anything that goes in your baby's mouth. Avoid hard foods and small round foods such as raisins or whole beans until your baby has molars for chewing. Never let your child run or play vigorously with anything in her mouth. A general rule for solids should be, the more teeth your child develops, the more capable she is of coping with firmer foods.

Here's a list of the most dangerous solid foods. Consider all of these choking hazards until your baby has molars to chew them:

Whole nuts (especially peanuts), until 3 years old

Popcorn (hulls are dangerous)

Raw carrots

Raw apples (watch out for peels)

Beans, unless mashed

The most important nutrient for your baby is proper fats. Breast milk is rich in the omega-3 fat DHA. Once your baby is eating solid foods, then she can begin a supplement of cod liver oil to ensure that adequate fats are supplying nerve and brain cells for their proper development. Give your baby 1/4 teaspoon cod liver oil for every 12 pounds of body weight.

When introducing solid foods, use fresh fruits and vegetables whenever possible. Cook them yourself. This is not as difficult as it may sound, and it is more nutritious and safer than using prepared baby food from jars. Organic is always best. It is not safe to feed an infant pesticides or fertilizer by-products (see page 21).

Baby food jars themselves contain a chemical that may be hazardous to a baby's health, regardless of the nutritional value of the product inside. This chemical is known to cause cancer, liver damage, and genetic modifications. Called semicarbazide, it is found in the plastic sealing gaskets of glass jars with metal lids. The chemical leaches into the foods contained in these jars. Although the amount of the chemical is small and researchers are unsure what risk, if any, this poses to babies, the presence of this substance should give parents cause for concern. Baby food had the highest concentration of any prepared foods tested by the European Food Safety Authority (check out the report at www.efsa.eu.int), the European equivalent of the FDA. This organization has called for the removal of the chemical from food jar gaskets. Besides the risk from this specific chemical exposure, jars of prepared baby food are lower in vitamin content than homemade food. And they're much more expensive.

The nutrient content of baby food products in jars may be considerably inferior to their freshly cooked counterparts. Nutrients in single-ingredient baby foods (first-stage foods) varies depending on the amount of water present in the jar. The carbohydrate content of first-stage foods is a measure of the amount of fruit or vegetable present compared to the amount of water. The brand with the highest carbohydrate content contains nearly 80 percent more carbohydrate than the brand with the least amount (Stallone and Jacobson, 1995). Second-stage and third-stage baby food jars contain a variety of fillers and sweeteners, including tapioca, sugar, corn syrup, and cornstarch, that can dramatically reduce the nutrient content of these foods. For example, bananas with tapioca and prunes with tapioca provide half or less the amount of nutrients of fresh bananas and prunes. The Heinz preparation with tapioca contains only 28 percent of the riboflavin, vitamin B_6, and potassium per ounce compared to the Heinz first-stage food without tapioca (Stallone and Jacobson, 1995). A typical "mixed vegetables" preparation by Gerber or Heinz contains three kinds of starch thickeners (wheat flour, oat flour, and potato solids or potato flour). Any amount of flour or starch will signify a nutritionally inferior product.

Commercial baby food is considerably more expensive than homemade baby food. Jars of sweet potatoes typically cost four times as much as homemade. Mashed bananas typically cost fifteen times as much. I do not recommend ever feeding your baby prepared jars of food. If you need to use these prepared foods (during unusual circumstances, such as traveling with your baby), only use organic products. Jars of organic food cost 25 percent more than the commercially grown products, but the difference is well worth the added cost.

I encourage parents to make their own baby food from organic fruits, vegetables, and meats whenever possible. Several excellent books provide detailed instructions for home preparation of foods for children age 5 months to 3 years; one of the best is *Super Baby Food* by Ruth Yaron. I agree with most of her preparation methods except for her recommendation to use a microwave oven. She also has an unnecessary hypervigilance about microbes, and she recommends the introduction of cereals at too young an age.

Parents can easily prepare their own applesauce, cooked pears, prunes, and vegetables. There are two options to puree cooked foods. Buy a small jar that screws onto the base of your blender. You should be able to find these through the website of your blender manufacturer. This will allow you to easily blend small portions of cooked fruits and vegetables. Use the water that you used to steam the vegetables or add water until your baby's food is the right consistency. The second option is to use a baby food grinder for preparing small amounts of food. This device has a hollow cylinder with a piston inside that pushes food up to the top to a hand-cranking grinder.

Do not microwave your baby's food or bottles. A Swiss study showed that changes in the blood of test subjects could be detected after eating foods cooked in microwave ovens. These changes included a decrease in all hemoglobin and cholesterol values, especially the ratio of HDL (high-density, or good cholesterol) to LDL (low-density, or bad cholesterol) values. Lymphocytes (white blood cells) showed a more distinct short-term decrease following the intake of microwaved food than after the intake of all the other variants. The variants of food consumed included raw milk, pasteurized milk, microwaved milk, raw organic vegetables, conventionally cooked vegetables, and the same vegetables cooked in a microwave oven. (Mercola, 1995). Dr. Lita Lee documents several studies that observed the formation of known carcinogens when vegetables, milk, meat, and grains were heated with microwaves. Russian researchers also reported a marked acceleration of structural degradation in microwave-heated foods leading to a decreased nutrient value of 60 to 90 percent in all foods tested (Lee, 1998).

Cereals and Disease

Many clinicians believe that early introduction of solids, especially grains, can trigger or cause eczema or other allergic disease in children later in life. This is not surprising since grains often stimulate allergic reactions and babies produce only small amounts of the enzyme amylase necessary for the digestion of grains until they reach age 1. Studies on the relationship of early introduction of solid foods and increased allergic reactions have resulted in conflicting results. Some studies show a relationship between eczema and early introduction of solids. One study found that infants who received solids at 8–12 weeks of age had a higher incidence of eczema by age 24 months (Forsyth et al., 1993). Another study found that preterm infants fed solids before 17 weeks post-term had a significantly higher risk of eczema by age 12 months post-term (Morgan et al., 2004). However, a different study, reported in the same pediatric journal issue, found no association between early introduction of solids and eczema or asthma (Zutavern et al., 2004).

Even more troubling is the association between childhood diabetes and the early introduction of cereals. Two studies published in the same issue of *JAMA* showed that early introduction of both rice cereal and gluten-containing foods (oats and wheat) into an infant's diet can stimulate the production of diabetes-associated autoantibodies. In these studies infants were chosen who had a family history of type 1 (child-onset) diabetes or who themselves carried the gene for diabetes.

Infants fed cereal prior to 3 months of age were four times as likely to develop these autoantibodies against pancreatic tissue compared to infants who delayed cereal introduction until 4–6 months of age. This does not mean that these children developed diabetes, but they did develop autoantibodies, which are associated with diabetes onset. What does this mean? Here is what the researchers concluded:

> A hypothesis could be explored about increased carbohydrate load in infancy and its impact on the pancreas and the immune system. . . . Carbohydrate loading in infancy may stimulate the pancreas to secrete more insulin, resulting in an increase in the expression of the autoantigens, which ultimately may increase the risk of islet cell [pancreas] destruction. (Ziegler et al., 2003)

Interestingly, if cereal introduction was delayed until age 7 months or older, the risk of autoantibody production was five times greater than for those infants where cereal was introduced at ages 4–6 months. The authors speculated that older babies were more likely to have a larger quantity of cereals than younger infants, thus increasing the carbohydrate load at initial cereal introduction in those children over 7 months old. Additionally, if a baby was still breastfeeding when cereals were introduced, the risk of autoantibody formation was reduced no matter what the age of the baby (Ziegler et al., 2003; Norris et al., 2003).

What is the message from these two studies? First, cereals can stimulate an autoimmune response in infants. Second, breastfeeding helps to protect the infant from the development of autoimmune reactions.

My advice is that anyone with a family history of childhood-onset diabetes should avoid giving an infant cereal, rice products, oats, or wheat. Babies will do fine without cereal if their mothers eat a diet rich in natural foods and adequate protein and take a high-quality vitamin/mineral supplement during pregnancy and while breastfeeding. Babies should be tested for anemia at 8 or 9 months of age because maternal iron stores typically wear out after six months (see page 160). Then solid food introduction should begin after age 5 or 6 months. Introduction of grains should be delayed in all infants until they are 12 months old and wheat should be delayed longer if there is a family history of food allergies or diabetes. And continue breastfeeding until well past the baby's first birthday because of breast milk's protective effect against many diseases.

The Danger of Nitrates

Many advisors caution parents about giving carrots, beets, and spinach to infants because of the high nitrate content of these vegetables. Nitrates are dangerous to infants because of an unusual set of circumstances. Infants have less stomach acid than adults, a situation that allows bacteria to grow in an infant's digestive system, converting nitrates into toxic nitrites. These nitrites then convert hemoglobin in red blood cells to methemoglobin, which cannot carry oxygen. Without oxygen babies can become asphyxiated, turning blue. That is how nitrates can cause the Blue Baby Syndrome. Babies older than 6 months usually have adequate stomach acid secretion to inhibit the bacteria that convert nitrate to its toxic form, although cases of the disease methemoglobinemia from eating vegetables (especially beets) have been recorded in older infants (Sanchez-Echaniz et al., 2001).

The highest concentrations of nitrates occurs in well water contaminated from fertilizer run-off, home prepared beets, carrots, and spinach. Nitrates in spinach can be converted to nitrites in the raw leaves even before they are consumed, and spinach consumption by infants has resulted in methemoglobinemia when the nitrite levels were high. Commercially prepared baby foods are tested for nitrate levels. If you feed your baby organic produce you can be assured that the nitrate levels will be relatively low. This is another excellent reason to wait six months before starting solid foods and to use only organic produce. Never give infants prepared meats made with nitrates or nitrites (hot dogs, bacon, salami, packaged turkey, and others).

Egg Yolks

Egg yolks supply cholesterol, which is needed for mental development. Remember, babies need fats. Organic, cage-free chicken's eggs will also contain omega-3 fatty acids that stimulate brain development. Feeding your baby one egg yolk every day from the age of 5–6 months will provide these essential nutrients, as well as vitamin A and amino acids.

You can either crumble a hard-boiled egg yolk and mix it with other foods, or scramble the yolk in a pan with coconut oil or butter. To separate the yolk from the white before cooking, place a funnel into a cup and crack the egg into the funnel. The white will drain out into the cup and the yolk will remain in the funnel. You can do the same thing with your hand if you like. Crack an egg into your palm and allow the white to drain out between your fingers into a bowl.

Do not give your baby raw eggs because of the slight chance of salmonella contamination. Soft-boiled egg yolks are fine as long as the eggs come from organic, cage-free sources.

ORDER OF SOLID FOOD INTRODUCTION

AGE 5–6 MONTHS (ALL PUREED OR MASHED FOODS):

Egg yolk (organic only)   Applesauce (organic)

Bananas   Stewed prunes

Steamed broccoli   Carrots (organic only)

Yams or sweet potatoes

AGE 7–9 MONTHS (SOFT OR MASHED FOODS):

Vegetable soups   Peas

Squash   Avocados

Peaches or nectarines

AGE 10–12 MONTHS (BEGIN TO GIVE SOFT SOLID PIECES):

Yogurt (whole-milk, organic, plain)   Butter

Chicken or turkey   Cooked vegetable pieces

Blueberries   Mangos

Papaya

AGE 12 MONTHS OR MORE (BEGIN TO GIVE PROTEIN AND CALCIUM SOURCES):

Oats, whole wheat breads and crackers   Cheese and cottage cheese

Whole egg   Cashew and almond butter

Oranges   Strawberries

Melons   Apples (peeled)

Grapes and raisins (seedless)   Corn

Spinach   Honey

Tahini

Feeding the Older Baby

As babies grow and eat a more varied diet, they will naturally express their likes and dislikes. Continue to offer babies new foods, even if they have refused them in the past. Often it will take many exposures for a baby or toddler to accept a new food. Babies usually eat all day, snacking on small amounts of solid foods and periodically tanking up on breast milk. Some babies will chow down to a big meal, but most are natural grazers. Let your baby guide you. Offer a variety of foods throughout the day once she is eating solids, and rest assured that she will get adequate nutrients if you use fresh fruits and vegetables, organic dairy products (preferably raw), and naturally raised meats. Avoid foods with added sugar, wheat (white) flour, and any flavorings or coloring agents. There is no reason to give your baby processed fruit juice. Pasteurization of juice destroys valuable enzymes and vitamins, and renders fruit juice little better than sugar water. Use a juicer at home and prepare your own apple juice or vegetable juices for your baby. Use sippy cups or a glass to feed your baby juice. Do not give your baby a bottle filled with juice because the sugar will remain in contact with her teeth for a longer period of time and promote bacterial growth and tooth decay.

A Note about Nutrition Books

In the appendix nutrition section are books that I recommend. Beware of nutrition books. They may contain erroneous and incorrect advice. The conventional stance on infant and child nutrition is often at odds with scientific evidence and good judgment. The commercial food industry is a powerful influence. Soy food manufacturers, baby food manufacturers, and formula companies may all attempt to lead astray unsuspecting parents. Even government committees make recommen-

---

FOODS THAT GET SPECIAL ATTENTION

HIGHLY ALLERGENIC: POTENTIALLY TOXIC:

Nuts and nut butters   Honey (until 12 months old)

Egg whites   Spinach (until 12 months old)

Milk   Soy milk

Kiwi   Tofu

Citrus (oranges, grapefruit)

Strawberries

Wheat

Corn

---

dations that defy good sense. The obsession with cholesterol and low-fat diets is especially insidious and destructive to the health of children. Low-fat diets are unsafe for children (see page 26). And the USDA food pyramid is simply wrong and misleading. Again, do not feed your baby soy products or soy formula (see page 51).

The table here outlines the appropriate order of solid food introduction. If a baby is not reacting to any foods, then parents can try moving foods up into an earlier time slot. If there is any family history of allergies, however, I suggest strict adherence to the schedule. If a baby does react to a particular food, stop it and wait. You can try reintroducing the food at a later date. The timing of the reintroduction will depend on the severity of the reaction and the type of food. You may want to discuss this with your baby's medical provider. Use organic foods whenever possible.

Teething

First colic, now teething. When will it stop? Some parents may wonder when they will finally see a full-time happy, contented baby. Other parents have no experience at all with fussiness. Some fussy-baby symptoms reflect the individual child's temperament. All children have their own styles of behavior, and these styles have been categorized. The behavior characteristics of babies that parents find most difficult are a high level of intensity of expression, difficulty adjusting to a new situation, and negative reactions. Easy babies tend to be mild in their emotional expression, adjust easily to change, and react positively to most stimuli.

Stress will intensify a child's difficult temperament reactions, and teething is a major stressor for some babies. Teething has the ability to intensify digestive disturbances, immune system reactions, and, of course, nervous system reactivity. Teething can be accompanied by diarrhea, cold symptoms, fevers, and lots of fussiness.

Babies at about 4 months will typically begin drooling and putting their fists into their mouths to chew on them. These expressions may be interpreted as teething by parents, and babies may experience discomfort as teeth move through the gums, but usually baby's teeth do not begin showing at the gum line until age 6 months or later. Some children will not get any teeth until well past their first birthday.

The purpose of teeth is to bite and chew food, though your baby may have other ideas. If your baby decides to use mom's nipple as a teething toy, take a firm tone and instruct her to stop. If you take away the nipple when she bites, she will soon get the idea that the breast is still just for sucking. The best teething device is a frozen banana. Peel a banana, slice it lengthwise, and cut it into pieces that your baby can hold. The combination of the cold on her gums, the sweetness, and the chewy texture holds her interest and soothes the discomfort. Another helpful device to have at home for both teething and feeding purposes is a mesh bag feeder. This device, called the Baby Safe Feeder, is essentially a ring with a small mesh bag attached that holds frozen fruit (mango, peach, grapes, and so on) and a handle for baby that screws onto the ring. You can find these online by searching for Baby Safe Feeder. I do not recommend plastic teething rings, or other plastic chew toys because of the chemicals that leach from the plastics. There is no need for teething gels, painkillers, or combination homeopathic tablets with teething. Usually a dose of home-opathic *Chamomilla* will help soothe your baby during fussy periods. The two Chinese herbal formulas Quiet Calm and Comfort Shen (made by Chinese Modular Solutions) can be ordered by your medical provider. These two formulas are also effective in calming a baby upset by teething.

The Role of Acute Illness

Newborns acquire antibodies to specific diseases from their mother's bloodstream while they reside in the uterus. These antibodies protect babies from pathogenic microbes in the environment. By the age of 6 months, however, these acquired antibodies typically disappear. Now susceptible to common viruses in the environment, your baby's own immune system will rally against them, developing its own antibody responses. During these episodes of immune response, your baby may develop symptoms of infection that consist of colds, fevers, coughs, and rashes. These challenges to your baby's system provide a form of immune exercise that builds immunity. This is a healthy process.

Babies who do not develop fevers in the first year of life have an increased risk of developing allergies and asthma (Calvani et al., 2002). Similarly, when antibiotics are given during the first year of life, children have an increased risk of allergy and asthma (Droste et al., 2000). Presumably, when the body's defenses against disease are not adequately stimulated early in life, a second defense system is activated that over-reacts to allergens. Researchers correlate this immune mechanism with two different types of white blood cells—one that responds to viruses and bacteria (TH1) and another that responds to parasites and releases histamine (TH2). If babies have not developed the TH1 white cells, then the excess of TH2 cells will stimulate allergies. When antibiotics deprive the baby of fighting off infections on her own, this same mechanism will occur and the immune system will be skewed in the direction of allergic responses.

When your baby gets sick with colds, fevers, and other infections, use natural methods of treatment that stimulate a healing response. Homeopathy, herbs, and nutritional supplements provide support to the body, help prevent complications of illness, and encourage the body's own defense system to marshal a vigorous response. Avoid using fever reducers (acetaminophen and ibuprofen) that prevent these responses, depriving the body of its healthy immune system reactions.

Anemia and Iron

Babies are born with a storehouse of iron acquired from their mother. Breast milk has only trace amounts of iron, but infants absorb iron at least ten times more efficiently from breast milk than from any other source. Around six months after birth, your baby's iron stores will start to become depleted. As babies begin to get iron from foods, their iron levels are replenished. There is a window, however, in the period 6–12 months of age when babies can become deficient in iron (anemia). Iron is the central atom in the hemoglobin molecule, the part of red blood

IRON SOURCES FOR BABIES

Liver (1 ounce)	2.5 mg
Beef (1 ounce)	1 mg
Kidney beans (1/8 cup)	2 mg
Tahini (1 tablespoon)	1 mg

cells that transports oxygen to cells in the body. Anemia causes a low level of hemoglobin and can lead to oxygen deprivation in sensitive areas of the brain, resulting in developmental delays.

All babies should be tested for anemia at around 9 months of age with a finger-stick blood test for hemoglobin. A hemoglobin level above 11 is normal. If your baby has a hemoglobin level below 11, then your medical provider may prescribe an iron supplement to boost the hemoglobin level. Iron drops can temporarily stain the teeth. Put the drops on the back of your baby's tongue and wipe her teeth with a piece of gauze to prevent staining. Give vitamin C with iron drops.

An excellent iron supplement for babies over 1 year of age is Floradix Iron and Herbs, which contains 7.5 mg iron in the form of ferrous gluconate per 2 teaspoons of the liquid. This iron supplement is derived from vegetarian sources and available at health food stores or online. Do not give it to babies younger than 12 months because it contains honey. Here are the ingredients of Floradix Iron and Herbs, from the label:

> Aqueous extract from Carrot, Nettle Wort, Spinach, Quitch roots, Angelica roots, Fennel; Ocean Kelp, African Mallow Blossom, Orange Peel; Juice Concentrates (pear, red grape, black currant, orange, blackberry, cherry, beetroot), Yeast (saccha-

romyces cerevisiae) Extract, Honey, Rosehip extract, Wheat
Germ Extract, Natural Flavor.

It is important for children to get iron in their diets. The best food
sources of iron are breast milk, liver, red meat, blackstrap molasses,
sesame seeds (tahini), and wheat germ. Iron from vegetable sources is better absorbed if combined with red meat, chicken, or turkey. All iron
sources are better absorbed in the presence of vitamin C. Children with
anemia should get vitamin C with meals. Use either a powdered form of
vitamin C (a buffered preparation such as calcium ascorbate works well
in juice or a smoothie) or vitamin C drops. Do not use chewable vitamin C. The acid in contact with molars can cause tooth decay. Milk can
interfere with iron absorption. If your baby is anemic, do not feed her
solids within twenty minutes of breastfeeding or formula. Spinach and
chard contain oxalic acid that interferes with iron absorption. The normal iron requirement is 0.5 mg per pound of body weight per day. Thus,
a 20-pound baby will need 10 mg of iron per day. An excellent iron supplement is a little frozen organic liver shredded into other pureed foods.
Cooking foods in an iron skillet will also increase the iron content.

CHAPTER 8

The Toddler

Your toddler is discovering the world at a phenomenal rate. Wake up in the morning and he has made leaps in his abilities you hardly imagined yesterday. Language skills, fine motor abilities, and an amazing capacity to absorb and understand the world around him all combine to make your child an endless source of wonder and surprises. His grasp of concepts and unrelenting questions may by turns entertain you or drive you to distraction. By the time your baby reaches the ripe age of 3, he has undoubtedly developed the reasoning and debate skills of a seasoned attorney.

Your toddler may present the biggest challenge you face as a parent. Not until the teenage years will you again face the relentless opposition to choices that seem obviously reasonable to you. Why does a toddler decide that only one particular spoon will work for his meal? Why does a 2-year-old ask for a sandwich and then throw it across the room because the crust is not cut off correctly? What happened to your agreeable baby, who seems to have been replaced by this tyrant?

It is the job of a 2-year-old to express and seek independence. But, at the same time, he is attached, reluctant to try new things, shy and suspicious of strangers, and often unwilling to let you leave. A mass of contradictions. This polarized state may send the toddler into a tizzy of tantrums and frustration, making it hard for you keep your equilibrium.

If you sometimes feel that you are on the losing end of a power struggle, rest assured that you have now joined the ranks of parents similarly reduced to the level of a 2-year-old as well.

Food and the Toddler

Young children need nutrient-dense foods. Their need for animal products is much greater than that of adults. Toddlers require fats in the form of butter, eggs, raw milk, cheese, meat, and coconut oil. Whole grains, soups, and fruit round out the diet of the toddler set.

You may find your agreeable 1-year-old getting more and more picky about foods as he grows. This selectivity reflects the natural progression of emotional development. Most children choose a certain set of foods, then switch to a new set, making it difficult to stay current on the latest favorites. Parents usually resort to a guessing game called, What would you like to eat today? Often the chosen few foods fall within a monochrome palette of pasta, cheese, bread, bananas, and apples—everything as white as possible. Don't worry. Soon your finicky toddler will discover a wider array of fruits, vegetables, and meats once again, but don't plan on a broad menu selection in the preschool years.

Toddlers eat snacks. They are natural grazers and not inclined to sit down to large meals. This is because their digestive systems are relatively weak and unable to metabolize and transform large amounts of food. Keep a steady supply of healthful snacks available, and continue to offer nutritious foods even if your preschooler has repeatedly refused them. Sooner or later he will try them again and find that he likes them. You may want to keep cut-up fruit in a bowl on a low table for him. Whole wheat crackers, cheese, a few vegetables, and dried fruit make for healthful snacks to leave in strategic places around the house. Children older than 3 can snack on nuts. Maintaining a steady blood sugar level in toddlers will help to avoid mood swings and meltdowns. When you travel in the car, take along a lunch box with an ice pack to keep snacks cool.

Oatmeal is the ideal cereal for children. Soak the oats overnight in a ratio of one part oats to one part water. Then add one part of water again and a pinch of salt prior to cooking the oats. Melt some butter on the hot oatmeal and add milk to increase the saturated fat and vitamin A content. Be aware that the grains in cold breakfast cereal from boxes are devitalized and nutritionally damaged.

Flakes, puffed cereals, and little O's are prepared under conditions of high temperatures and pressures, both of which cause rancidity and destruction of vitamins and amino acids. In one study of rats fed a diet of puffed wheat and water with added vitamins and minerals, the rats died in two weeks. Rats fed the same diet using whole wheat instead of puffed wheat lived for one year. This suggested that something about the processing of the wheat actually created toxins that killed the rats because the group that received water and nutrients but no food lived for eight weeks (Stitt, 1983).

Avoid giving your toddler commercial fruit juices, which are devoid of nutritional value. Make juices yourself from fruits and vegetables. Think of pasteurized, bottled juices as sugar water. The most nutritious drink for your children is raw milk (see page 39). Drinks made from soy and rice have high levels of phytates that disturb mineral absorption.

Children seem to universally accept peanut butter, and although it will contribute to the omega-6 fat portion of your child's diet, peanuts also represent a good source of protein. Use organic peanut butter, preferably from Valencia peanuts that tend to have less mold. Many organic peanut butter manufacturers state that they do test for molds and aflatoxin, a natural carcinogen contained in the mold that grows on peanuts. Beware of peanut butters with added partially hydrogenated oils. Peanut allergy is particularly common. Consult with your child's medical provider about the safe age to introduce peanuts into the diet. Delay giving peanuts until your child is at least 2 years old and then begin slowly, testing as you would with the introduction of any potential allergen. Tahini, made from sesame seeds, is a safe alternative, and a valuable source of calcium. Other nuts are equally nutritious, including almonds and cashews. Nut butters are a concentrated and valuable addition to the diet of older children.

Preschoolers have a natural affinity for sweet foods, so the longer you can postpone the inevitable exposure to sugar-filled desserts, the better off your child will be. Make cookies and baked foods at home with whole grains and eggs and fruits, with limited amounts of sweeteners.

Safety

Keeping a toddler safe is a full-time job. Babyproofing your home is the first step in guaranteeing that your baby will not suffer injury from household products and lurking dangers.

A variety of devices available at your local hardware store will provide the tools to make your home safe. Install cabinet locks everywhere your baby can reach—under the sinks, into spice cabinets or cupboards filled with pots, pans, and dishes. Remove poisons from low cabinets and put them high up, out of reach. Consider replacing commercial cleaning products with natural, nontoxic cleaners, or use a solution of vinegar and water for most clean-up jobs. Fill electrical outlets with plastic inserts and cover plugs with outlet cover boxes. Get baby locks for the toilet, and consider putting one on the refrigerator. Place a cover device over the range controls. Put gates at the top and bottom of stairways. Never allow electrical cords to hang within baby's reach—for example, when ironing clothes. Crawl around on the floor yourself and imagine what your baby could get into, pull over, or climb on. Fix free-standing cabinets and bookcases to the walls. I have seen a climbing baby pull down an entire shelf system and a television on top of himself. Be vigilant about doors that open to the front or back yards or outer hallways. Never leave a small child unattended in a bath or wading pool. Children can drown in a few inches of water. Do not use walkers with wheels. They can be easily tipped, trapping your baby. But remember: The fewer restraining devices, the better. Your baby will profit from the freedom to explore and not from the constraints of bouncers and playpens.

Toilet Training

Let your child guide the potty training plan. Follow your child's lead. Some girls are ready to use the potty by 18 months. Most boys have no interest until they reach age 3. Personality, temperament, and season of the year all affect the timing of that glorious day when you are free of diapers. If your toddler is pointing to his diaper when he pees, then you can begin to coax him to use the potty instead. During the summer months you can leave your baby's diaper off and encourage him to pee outside or let you know when the urge strikes. Many children will be interested in the potty for a while, then decide it's not worth the effort.

If your child attends a preschool program, there may be a high expectation to use the toilet and be diaper-less. Preschoolers have a tendency to conform to the rules outside the home but resist any pressure within the home. Avoid pressure tactics or forceful efforts to encourage potty use.

Keep a special potty available, and suggest that your child can use it. Read some picture books about potties, but don't force the issue. Try not to give the impression that your child's decision to use the potty would probably relieve and please you more than anything. As with all your child's accomplishments, give plenty of positive reinforcement when he actually uses the potty for its intended purpose.

Tantrums

Brace yourself. What you have heard about 2-year-olds is true. And 3-year-olds. Some children are bossy, some downright dictatorial. Others give true meaning to the phrase "throwing tantrums." Whether your child is merely rambunctious, out of control, shriekingly loud, or a sheer terror, there is help. Several forms of natural treatment have the ability to mitigate the worst of the temper fits and bring your child into a more harmonious emotional balance.

Constitutional homeopathy has the most dramatic curative effect on the emotional disturbances of the preschool years, compared to any other treatment. Homeopathic medicine has a clearly delineated and described set of medicines appropriate for the syndrome of the emotionally distraught toddler or preschooler. Parents would do well to consult a trained and experienced homeopath when children seem overwhelmed by their emotions and the developmental demands of this age. Often a single dose of the correct constitutional medicine will work like magic to bring a child back into a state of natural equilibrium. Like any deep-acting homeopathic treatment, the medicine must be chosen that fits the child's symptom expression, personality, and general characteristics of physiology. A wide range of medicines can be prescribed for this situation, and the homeopath must carefully choose between them by observing the symptoms, hearing about them, and discerning the real motivation and cause for the behaviors in that child. A variety of prescribing methods are available to the homeopath to bring about a cure, including the prescription of daily doses of a liquid or pellet preparation of the medicine.

A DHA supplement (fish oil or algae sourced) can have striking effects to ease behavior and emotions. Chinese herbs can also alleviate the drama of these symptoms.

Try to avoid confrontations with a reluctant preschooler. Offer choices rather than giving orders. Even if it doesn't work you may be able to avoid complete rebellion. Try not saying no. The more you say no, the more likely you are to hear it shouted right back at you. It's hard not to lose your temper at times, but remember that the carpet, or the car finish, or the broken glass mean nothing compared to your relationship with your child.

Try to think like your child: Being 2 is frustrating. You know what you want, and often you know how to get it, but it is difficult to make yourself understood. When your language skills do not match your great ideas, then it is easy to get frustrated and lose your temper. When your just-developing fine motor skills do not allow you to create the perfect picture you have in mind, then it may be time to start throwing things across the room or striking out at the closest object in sight—Mommy.

Never hit your child. Never shake your child. If you must confine him to some safe area, do it. Remove him physically from any space that is unsafe when he pitches a fit. Moving your child out of the area that stimulated the meltdown will tend to defuse the behavior. Take him outside if possible. Young children are easily distracted. Use that knowledge to your advantage. Remember that your child has nothing better to do than try to get an emotional reaction from you. Attention, either positive or negative, is interesting to a 2-year-old who has difficulty understanding cause and effect. If you have reached your limit, call a friend, or start counting until you calm down. Give yourself a time-out, not your child. Time-outs can defuse the situation, but they tend to cause resentment in children. If you put your child into a corner or on a chair and instruct him to think about what he has done, what he may be thinking is, *I hate you, I hate you.*

Another word about "no." Of all the tools your child has for relationships, "no" is one of the most useful. No is a very safe space for kids.

When you ask them a question, if they say yes, they are committed, but if they say no, then they have bought some time to consider the issue. Kids realize they can always change their minds. Eventually, no becomes the automatic response. For many kids, the watchword *Don't agree to anything* serves them well. Parents are constantly trying to trick children. Reverse psychology is rampant, and offering equally irksome choices to manipulate a response is a common parental tactic. No wonder kids adopt a cautious, suspicious attitude. How else to cope with adults than to say no and thereby hold your ground? Learn to appreciate your child's resourcefulness, persistence, and strategizing techniques. Ignore the negativity and your relationship will prosper.

Frequent Colds and Ear Infections

The most common reason for doctor visits among 1- to 3-year-olds is ear infections. And pediatricians expect six to eight colds a year. This pattern of illness is completely avoidable and easily cured with the correct treatment. The causes of frequent illnesses among preschoolers are an assault on the immune system by vaccines and antibiotics, and an inappropriate diet. Weakened immune systems in this age group are responsible for the rampant plague of repeated ear infections with persistent fluid in the middle ear, swollen adenoids, constant congested nose with allergies and sinus infections, and the escalating incidence of asthma. These children consume significant amounts of drugs and suffer inordinate numbers of surgeries for ear tube placement and adenoid removal. Antibiotics promote recurrent infections. They weaken immune function, create bacterial resistance, and destroy the valuable protective bacteria that help control pathogens. Much safer alternatives exist.

The first step in treatment is to strengthen the immune system and avoid foods that aggravate the condition. Extended breastfeeding pre-

FRUSTRATING EAR PROBLEMS: A CASE HISTORY

Shannon's mom, Lisa, had reached the end of her rope. She thought she always did the right thing—at least she tried. Natural childbirth, organic foods, breastfeeding, no drugs. She gave in when Shannon had an earache. On a 1-to-10 scale, the pediatrician said the eardrum was a bright red 8, and she relented. After the antibiotics and Shannon's return to preschool, within two weeks another earache. Back to the doctor. More antibiotics. Two months later Shannon still had fluid in her ears. "That's pretty typical," the doctor said. "Let's send her to an ENT specialist." Lisa suspected the pediatrician just didn't want to hassle with her about giving more antibiotics, because the ENT gave her two choices, maintenance antibiotics or tubes in the ears. Lisa was horrified at the idea of surgery, so she began her search. There must be something more natural than those options. She called everyone she knew who was into natural forms of treatment, organic foods, or La Leche League. The name of a holistic doctor kept coming up. Lisa made an appointment.

The plan sounded too simple—a homeopathic medicine given only one time. "Not every day?" Lisa asked. The rest sounded easy too. Stop dairy products for now. Take a Chinese herbal formula that will decrease the size of her adenoids and another that will decrease the congestion and inflammation in her ears. And no more antibiotics. Call if she has any acute illnesses. See me in a month.

Within a week Shannon's hearing improved. She no longer said "what" all the time. Within three weeks she stopped snoring. Coincidental things occurred. Her mood improved, she slept better, she began talking more, and her appetite returned to normal. The teachers remarked that Shannon had become livelier at preschool. When Lisa brought Shannon back to the new doctor, no more fluid. He gave Shannon a cartoon sticker as a prize and pronounced her well on the way to being cured.

vents allergies, asthma, and infections. Supplements that promote healthy immune function include DHA from fish oil or algae sources, bovine colostrum, vitamin A, D, and C, probiotics (*bifidus* in breastfeeding babies and acidophilus in older children), and zinc polynicotinate. Several Chinese herbal formulas also build a strong immune system. Consult a holistic pediatric practitioner for advice about using these supplements to overcome weakened resistance to illness and develop optimum immune function in your child.

The second step to get these kids healthy is to treat them with medicines capable of initiating a healing response that results in cure. Constitutional homeopathic treatment by a knowledgeable practitioner is the most effective, most direct, and simplest method of curing the susceptibility to repeated infections. Chiropractic adjustments and Chinese herbal constitutional treatment can also create a healthy balance and stimulate immune function to overcome these cyclic patterns of illness and suppressive drug treatment.

CHAPTER 9

The School-Age Child

Once your child enters school, a whole new world opens before you. Preschool is mostly play and socializing, with some problem solving and a few pre-reading skills possibly thrown into the mix. Kindergartens in most communities now are quickly getting to the business of letters, numbers, and beginning readers. In first grade, children are expected to read. From there the road gets more difficult and children have many stresses to maneuver. At the same time, most kids are expected to pursue extracurricular exercise in the form of sports teams or dance classes. Any musical training is also primarily accomplished outside school hours.

Children need to experiment and discover their areas of interest and talents. All children should become experts in the subject areas that match their natural affinities. Children learn best when they feel compelled by the subject. They will seek out solutions to problems when the subject inspires them. As they gain expertise, they will also gain confidence and experience personal rewards for learning. Fortunately, our culture highly values and rewards the attainment of expertise in a wide range of subjects. Unfortunately for some children, particular subjects are more highly valued in our culture than others. Language and math are very highly regarded and rewarded on a daily basis. Children who excel in music, body intelligence, or spatial intelligence do not receive the same level of positive feedback. Sometimes these skills are never recognized or tapped at all. Similarly, children who have difficulty with language or math suffer under a significant disadvantage.

Parents are the managers of their child's educational experience and academic career. Teachers come and go. Schools change. Parents are the only consistent source of support for children in their growth and development through the years of early education. It is the job of a parent to monitor a child's progress in school, acknowledge achievements, and recognize difficulties. Parents must learn to understand their child's unique and individual style of learning. This is not always easy because many complex issues are involved in learning styles, including a child's temperament or behavioral style, attention skills, and the basic building blocks of learning functions. The more parents understand and know about their child's style of learning, the better equipped they will be to guide her toward achieving her highest potential. Parents who know their child well will be able to play to her strengths, encouraging success by continually presenting learning materials, explanations, and advice through the most effective channels for that individual child. For example, if your child is a strong visual learner but easily distracted, you can design a study environment with minimal distractions, present visual learning materials that will encourage her most effective means of achievement, and suggest that she always highlight textbooks and write out summaries of text passages she reads. Parents must also recognize when help is needed for learning difficulties and make decisions about how to get tutoring and remedial services either within or outside of the school. Several sections of this chapter are therefore devoted to developing an understanding of your child's learning functions and style.

Stresses of peer groups and high expectations can cause difficulty for school-age children. After fifth grade, peer groups begin to take on an ever increasing role for children. Friendships, loyalties, and cliques all take up a great deal of energy for most children when maneuvering through the social strata of grade school. For boys, a primary factor in the development of both self-confidence and acceptance by peers is the level of proficiency at sports. For girls, interpersonal skills may be the deciding factor between acceptance and rejection by a peer group. Parents may value and praise academic achievement and prowess, or even musical attainments, but peers are interested in how children relate within the pack.

Homeschooled children have a special advantage because many of the peer and societal stresses related to performance never come into play. Children who do not attend institutes of formal education can proceed at their own pace with daily one-on-one personal attention. They can progress quickly through material that they find easy, spend more time on compelling subjects, and work without fear of embarrassment on building skills in weaker areas of learning. Homeschooled children tend to do very well in higher education settings because of the advantages that an individually designed learning program affords them.

Nutrition and School Lunches

It is crucial for a child's health and success in academic areas to maintain a high level of nutrition. School is more demanding for children than ever before, and their energy will flag, their attention and concentration will suffer, and their immune systems will become depleted if their nutritional support is not excellent. However, even for parents committed to feeding their children the best possible diets, breakfast and lunch remain difficult areas to negotiate with kids.

Breakfast is often described as the most important meal, but it usually gets little attention and poor scores for nutrients. Most older children eat packaged cereal for breakfast and snacks loaded with sugar and deficient in nutrients. Puffed cereal, flakes, and O's are all processed with significant heat and pressure, both of which cause rancidity and destroy nutrients (see page 165).

The easiest way to get kids started on the right foot in the morning is to feed them eggs, oatmeal soaked overnight, whole wheat products, and fresh fruit. Cook the eggs in butter or coconut oil. French toast or pancakes made with eggs and whole wheat are also good variations. Soaking the wheat overnight in yogurt, buttermilk, or water with lemon juice will break down irritating proteins and release nutrients. Appropriate toppings are apple butter, pure fruit spreads, or organic pure maple syrup. Do not use corn syrup substitutes. Don't forget the butter to increase the saturated fats in your children's diets. For some excellent recipes, see *Nourishing Traditions* by Sally Fallon and Mary Enig. If children will drink a smoothie, you can use fruit, raw cow's milk, and some powdered supplements of colostrum, vitamin C, and zinc to bolster immune function. Children can eat other protein sources also, including organic bacon or sausage, or leftover chicken.

Lunches served at most schools are notoriously unhealthful. Ingredients of a typical school lunch include trans fats, nitrates, sugar, corn syrup, artificial colors and flavors, and lots of white flour. A few elementary schools around the country have developed organic lunch programs. You can work to establish an organic garden and organic food program at your child's school and get involved with other groups that are pursuing better food programs in schools. The Marin Food Systems Project has resources for school groups to develop better school food policies (check out www.eecom.net/projects_school_actionguide.htm). Stonyfield Farm yogurt company has developed a blueprint for model school district legislation to bring more healthful foods into schools (www.stonyfield.com/MenuForChange/index.cfm). In the meantime, encourage your children to bring lunch from home.

Here are some lunchbox ideas. Chicken or turkey sandwiches made with whole wheat bread, peanut butter, cut-up fruit and raw vegetables, cheese, chicken drumsticks, sushi, cole slaw, potato salad, fruit bars, and even a thermos of homemade soup. For some great ideas about lunchbox items for your kids, see *The School Lunchbox Cookbook* by Miriam Jacobs.

If you establish good eating habits during the elementary school years, they will probably persist through the teenage years. The main problems with children's diets are excessive sugar consumption, the universal presence of corn syrup, snacking on chips, eating in front of the television, and an inadequate consumption of fresh fruits and vegetables. Children at this age need to continue supplementing their diets with omega-3 fats (fish oil) because of the protective effect they provide for brain functions and the immune system.

Allergies and Asthma

Allergic conditions can begin at any age. Infants can develop eczema soon after birth. Babies can also suffer from asthmatic reactions to viruses, with chronic coughs and/or wheezing following colds. Preschoolers may develop sensitivity to milk and chronic sinus congestion or ear problems. It is during the ages 5 through 10, however, that allergies and asthma become especially prevalent. Children at this age develop seasonal hay fever attacks and asthmatic reactions to animals, dust mites, and plants. Asthma may also manifest as exercise-induced wheezing when children begin playing sports (soccer, basketball, swimming) that challenge their endurance.

Allergies affect about 38 percent of all Americans, and about 5 percent of the U.S. population has asthma. The highest proportion of asthma is among children age 5 to 14, a total of 5 million children. Childhood asthma has increased by more than 40 percent since 1980. In other parts of the world, the numbers are even higher. In Western Europe as a whole, asthma cases have doubled in the last ten years, according to the UCB Institute of Allergy in Belgium. "The prevalence of asthma in children can be as high as 30 percent in certain populations," explained Professor Romain Pauwels, Chairman of the Global Initiative for Asthma (GINA). "In Australia, for example, one child in six under the age of 16 is affected today. Experts are struggling to understand why rates worldwide are, on average, rising by 50 percent every decade."

Many researchers have looked at the growing number of childhood vaccines as a likely cause of the rise in childhood asthma. Several clinical studies have confirmed an association between vaccination and asthma. A team of New Zealand researchers followed 1,265 children born in 1977. Of the children who were vaccinated, 23 percent had asthma episodes. A total of 23 children did not receive the DTP vaccines, and none of them developed asthma (Kemp et al., 1997). A study in Great Britain produced similar findings that associated asthma with the pertussis vaccine. In that study, 243 children received the vaccine and 26 of them later developed asthma (10.7 percent), compared to only 4 of the 203 children who had never received the pertussis vaccine (2 percent). Additionally, of the 91 children who received no vaccines at all, only one had asthma. Therefore, the risk of developing asthma was about 1 percent in children receiving no vaccines and 11 percent for those children who received vaccines, including pertussis (Odent et al., 1994). A third study was conducted in the U.S. from data in the National Health and Nutrition Examination Survey of infants through adolescents aged 16. Data showed that children vaccinated with DTP or tetanus were twice as likely to develop asthma, compared to unvaccinated children (Hurwitz and Morgenstern, 2000).

Medications given to children early in life also have a significant effect on the incidence of asthma. Children given antibiotics or acetaminophen (Tylenol) at some time prior to age 4 were nearly twice as likely to develop asthma, compared to a control group (Cohet et al., 2004). One group of researchers discovered a possible cause for the development of asthma as a consequence of antibiotic use. Mice given antibiotics developed an alteration of intestinal bacteria and an increase in the growth of intestinal yeast. These mice developed typical allergic responses in the lungs when they were exposed to mold spores. Mice that did not receive antibiotics did not experience the allergic reactions (Noverr et al., 2004).

Low income level has also proven to be associated with childhood asthma. In a study undertaken by the Harlem Children's Zone, more than 2,000 children were tested for asthma. All children under 13 who lived within a twenty-four-square block area of Central Harlem were tested, and 26 percent had evidence of asthma, five times the national average. Clearly, healthful nutrition is an important deterrent to the development of asthma in children.

The dramatic increase in childhood allergies and asthma has resulted in an equally alarming number of drug-dependent children. Parents have become dismayed at the inadequacies and dangers of conventional drug treatment for asthma. Most children with asthma are prescribed steroid inhalers with their attendant dangers of growth suppression and immune system depletion. Allergy drug recalls, deaths associated with asthma drugs, and the dire consequences of children on steroids have stimulated millions of parents to find alternatives. All of these drugs merely relieve symptoms for a few hours with no expectation of overall improvement. Effective conventional treatment for young children with allergies is virtually nonexistent.

The solution to allergic and asthmatic conditions lies in the realm of holistic medical care. Allergies can be significantly improved, and even cured, with holistic treatment. Homeopathic constitutional medicine is the most profound and direct way to stimulate a healing reaction and overcome immune system susceptibilities. Children's immune mechanisms can also be strengthened using a combination of nutritional supplements and Chinese herbal treatment. Treating asthma with holistic approaches can be complex and needs to be carefully managed— children cannot stop their medications suddenly. A number of safe and effective herbal formulas exist that can control asthma in children and simultaneously strengthen the immune system to prevent further attacks. The Chinese Modular Solutions formulas Open Air, Deep Breath, and Chest Relief, all developed for pediatric use, are especially effective in managing asthma without drugs.

Nutritional support for asthma is especially important, including adequate supplies of vitamins A, C, D, and E, colostrum, magnesium, and an omega-3 supplement. Several important herbal formulations can also help bolster immunity in older children, especially those combinations that include the immune stimulating mushrooms (maitake, reishi, grifola, polyporus, tremella).

Other treatment methods that can improve lung function and create a healthy balance in the body for energy to flow properly include acupuncture, and chiropractic and osteopathic manipulation.

Finally, the emotional and energetic component of asthma treatment should not be neglected. The field of psycho-neuro-immunology has revealed the important connection between emotions and the immune system. Self-regulation techniques that develop a relaxation state include guided imagery, biofeedback, and simple deep abdominal breathing. These methods can help prevent asthma reactions. Children proficient in these skills can also relieve asthmatic symptoms when they occur. One of the primary mechanisms of asthma is the constriction of smooth muscle fibers that encircle the airway tubes. When the mind is calm, when skeletal muscles are relaxed, and when breathing is deep and reg-

BREATHING AGAIN: A CASE HISTORY

Kayley is a fun-loving, friendly, and talkative first-grader. She likes Barbies and art projects and playing with her dog. Unfortunately, Kayley has some health problems that interfere with her life and play. She gets out of breath and coughs when she plays soccer. If she catches a cold it will quickly settle into nightly coughing spells that often worsen and turn into wheezing episodes. Twice, they have gotten so bad that she landed in the emergency room where the doctors used inhaled drugs to restore her breathing and then sent her home with a prescription for oral, systemic steroids.

The allergist prescribed an inhaled steroid for Kayley to use every day and a second bronchodilator drug for Kayley to take before exercise and whenever she developed cough or wheezing. Kayley's mother was not especially happy with the doctor's pronouncement that Kayley required continuous drug treatment, nor did she appreciate the side effects. The drugs made Kayley hyper. So began the search for alternatives to the standard drug approach for Kayley's asthma.

When I first saw Kayley, she still had a chronic dry, tight cough despite the drug treatment. Since Kayley was in no acute distress and the drugs were not preventing or curing her symptoms anyway, we decided to replace the daily drug regimen with Chinese herbs and put Kayley on a program of immune enhancing supplements. I prescribed a liquid extract of herbs formulated for children (Deep Breath by Chinese Modular Solutions) and a similar formula for acute episodes of cough or wheezing (Open Air). She received one dose of a constitutional homeopathic medicine, *Natrum-sulphuricum* (1M strength).

Kayley needed help getting through her wintertime colds. Echinacea, vitamin C, herbs, and homeopathic treatment prevented the downward spiral that used to occur with her acute illnesses. Mild allergic rashes improved with supportive treatment. She never took steroids again, and she continued to excel at soccer and gymnastics. Her mother was frankly amazed at the new level of Kayley's resilience when she caught a cold. Chronic coughing was no longer a problem, and Kayley stopped identifying herself as an asthmatic.

ular, these muscles that constrict air flow will also relax and allow children to breathe more freely. Regular exercise, swimming, and dance training have also been shown to increase lung capacity and reduce asthma episodes.

This holistic approach to asthma will strengthen the immune system and lung function, prevent the airway inflammation characteristic of asthma, relieve the muscle constriction that impairs breathing, decrease mucus production in airways, and create a balanced energy flow that allows the lungs to do their job without impairment.

Bedwetting

Most children remain dry at night by the time they are 4. However, a small percentage of children will continue to wet the bed until they are 10–12 years old. By age 12 only 2 percent of children continue to wet their beds. Bedwetting is hereditary. It is usually due to a delay in the development of the hormone that prevents the bladder from filling during the night. Persistent bedwetting is usually not due to emotional causes, but a child who was dry for an extended period may respond to either physical or emotional stress by reverting to wetting the bed. A bladder infection or another physical illness can also cause nighttime or daytime accidents. Children who wet the bed do not have any different sleep patterns or brainwave signals than other children. Bedwetting can be a nuisance, an embarrassment, and a deterrent to social activities like sleep-overs, but children should be told that it always goes away sooner or later on its own. Parents should maintain a positive and reassuring attitude toward this problem.

Children 6 or older who are motivated to stop wetting the bed can do a program of buzzer training. This involves wearing a buzzer at night with a sensor attached to the underwear. When the sensor becomes slightly wet, the buzzer will wake the child and the parents. Everyone must get up, change the underwear and the bedding if it is wet, reattach the sensor, and then go back to bed. This requires effort and commitment on the part of children and parents. The program trains the child to waken at the first sign of leaking urine. If this nighttime training is combined with conditioning training during the day, the success rate is higher. Parents do this by asking the child to pee in the toilet and then setting off the buzzer. The child stops the flow of urine when she hears the buzzer. This presumably conditions the child to stop urinating in the night if the buzzer sounds. My experience is that any concerted attention that children apply to bedwetting will help to stop it. Alarm buzzers can be purchased online at www.bedwettingstore.com.

Homeopathy has been successful in ending bedwetting. This typically requires the proper constitutional homeopathic medicine, rather than a specific medicine for bedwetting itself.

Temperament Styles

Temperament refers to specific aspects of behavioral styles in children. Parents can develop more tolerance and more appropriate reactions if they understand their child's temperament style. All parents already know their children and can predict their reactions in various situations that they may find stressful. As parents, you already have methods for avoiding reactions that you find difficult to manage. If your daughter becomes upset at transitions, you learn to give her warnings, for example, that she will need to stop playing soon because it will be time for bed. Or, if your son has a high activity level, you learn to develop times for quiet play like reading to settle him down. Temperament characteristics are present in babies, and your child's particular temperament style will persist throughout his or her life.

Parents find some behaviors "easy," and other behaviors "difficult" to handle. For that reason clinical researchers have described the temperament styles in four categories: easy, difficult, slow-to-warm-up, and inflexible.

The behavioral styles that parents find easy to negotiate are a mild disposition and positive responses. These children have a low level of intensity and are engaging, often smiling, and agreeable. Parents and teachers find them pleasant and remarkably adaptable. They tend to get a lot of positive reinforcement because they aim to please.

By contrast, difficult behaviors for parents include a high level of intensity, negative reactions, and hard transitions. These children get excited easily, creating dramatic scenes, and they have critical, negative responses when offered choices. They take a while to get used to new situations, and have difficulty adjusting to a change so that transitions from one activity to another are stressful. Parents of these children can become testy, anticipating negative reactions and becoming guarded and negative themselves in response. Parents of "difficult" children find themselves confronting their own anger and tolerance levels. These children can be especially disruptive to families, especially if they are very active and intense. For this reason they get an inordinate amount of negative feedback. Their parents need to develop a thick skin so that these children can express themselves without being constantly reprimanded. The challenge for these parents is to channel their child's excitement and enthusiasm into realms that will produce positive results and build their self-esteem. An obvious repository for all of this kinetic energy is sports, but these children can also become experts in a wide range of fields from mechanics to rock music, depending on their proclivities. The high intensity level of these children can serve them well when they become excited about a particular subject and decide to master a technique of, say, snowboarding or model building or computer science.

Parents of these kids often seek help in developing management strategies from teachers, therapists, and self-help books. An entire industry
of books has been dedicated to the difficult or high-need child. Some of
these books are excellent resources full of strategies for parents to maintain their equilibrium, establish limits, and provide loving discipline so
that these children can both express their natural exuberance and learn
self-control. See the appendix for suggestions.

Parents of these children in the high-intensity realm with other temperament qualities that parents find difficult can get help from natural
treatment methods. Homeopathy is the premier treatment for stabilizing mood and bringing the high activity level, intensity, and negativity
into a more even realm. Homeopathic treatment will not change a child's
personality, but it will create a healthier emotional balance and bring
more self-control skills into play. Chinese herbs provide significant tools
for creating balance and relieving the extremes of emotional expression. Chiropractic treatment is often helpful for readjusting the nervous system involvement in these children, which can aggravate the
temperament characteristics and create extreme behavioral patterns.
Keeping these children's blood sugar at an even level throughout the
day is also helpful in avoiding the highs and lows that are often expressed
with great intensity. These children do well if they eat frequent small
meals and avoid foods with high sugar content and artificial stimulants.
They should especially avoid aspartame, artificial flavors and colors,
high-fructose corn syrup, and sugar-laden cereals, candy, and baked
products. Eating protein foods throughout the day also has a blood sugar
stabilizing effect. Finally, all of these children should be taking an omega-
3 fat supplement (see page 30).

Shy, cautious children are characterized as slow-to-warm-up. They
tend to observe new situations before participating. They find new places
and unfamiliar activities overwhelming. They tend to withdraw at first

THE TEMPERAMENT STYLES

THE EASY CHILD

| Mild intensity | Positive responses | Adaptable | Friendly |

THE DIFFICULT CHILD

| Intense | Negative responses | Slow to adapt | Withdraws |

SLOW-TO-WARM-UP

| Mild intensity | Negative responses | Slow to adapt | Withdraws |

INFLEXIBLE

| High intensity | Low distractibility | Slow to adapt |

when they encounter a new setting, class, or extracurricular activity. They may be curious and excited to try a new activity, but then intimidated by the reality of it once they participate, and then want to leave. Parents of these children need to learn patience. They also need to anticipate this reaction by staying nearby in new settings and allowing their child to observe for a while before joining the group at, say, ballet class, gymnastics, the soccer team, or swim lessons. These children need to make agreements that they will try something for a few classes before they quit. Once they get into the flow of the class, they are usually fine. Parents can prepare these children for a new grade at school by visiting the classroom and the teacher before the start of the school year. Reading books about an activity or viewing a video can help familiarize children with a new activity.

Parents may have certain expectations about their child's temperament that may or may not fit the way things turn out to be. It is part of the art of parenthood to modify our responses to our children's indi-vidual styles. What works for one child in the family may not be effec-tive for another, and when parents understand their child's reactions they can anticipate problems and build settings where the most har-monious result will occur. We can't expect that a slow-to-warm-up child will jump into a new class with exuberant enthusiasm, and we can't expect that an intense, active, and spirited child will sit still for long periods of time without hands-on explorative activities. The con-cept of Goodness of Fit has been applied to the creation of a setting where a child will flourish. Recognize the individual style of your child's behavior and then evaluate the activity, school, teacher, or class that will best fit your child's interests and temperament style. This includes evaluating potential teachers' personal styles through an interview or soliciting the experience of other parents to determine the best fit of their personality with what you know of your child's nature. Apply-ing temperament models in this way will help children achieve their potential and move through the school years smoothly, avoiding frus-tration, conflict, and injuries to self-esteem.

Attention

Attention and attentiveness are somewhat paradoxical when viewed by adults. We expect children to pay attention. We expect them to be alert to subtle differences in similar written statements and visual pre-sentations, carefully noting mistakes and inconsistencies. We expect them to sit still for extended periods of time, applying themselves qui-etly and diligently to written materials. Distractibility and impulsiveness would seem to interfere with these skills that require focus and concen-tration. We also encourage them to excel at sports, which often require them to continually scan their environment, take quick evasive action, and maintain a high level of constant motion and aggressive behavior. Children with strong drives who trust their instincts and impulses receive praise and positive reinforcement on the playing field, but are frequently reprimanded in the classroom. We also encourage children to be inventive and creative, traits that depend on spontaneity and impulsive hunches. It's a lot to ask, and often a confusing message for kids.

Consider the advantages of sensory vigilance, distractibility, and ceaseless activity for animals in the wild. A bird whose fitful attention diverts quickly from one moving object to another is likely to avoid being someone's dinner. Consider the survival capabilities of a hyperactive monkey constantly scanning the environment for predators compared to his lethargic and passive sibling. The studious, methodical monkey may discover survival strategies that far exceed those of his hyperactive cousin— but only if he lives long enough. Most children are not concerned with survival. Individual attention styles vary, and the child who has persistent focus, flexibility of thinking, and discernment for salient detail is at a distinct advantage in the academic jungle. Restless, energetic, future-directed behaviors can build a corporate superstar, but these qualities earn your typical 10-year-old boy the label of hyperactive, or of actually having an attention disorder.

Attention as an issue has become a focus for our culture in recent years. In fact, there is now an entire industry devoted to attention problems with departments in university medical centers and their affiliated programs dedicated to treating this disorder. Children are labeled with the disorder, the pharmaceutical industry supports research on the various corresponding drugs, scholarly books are written on the subject, parent support groups are formed, catalogs of educational materials are published specific to this disease, and regular conferences are held on the disorder.

My fundamental assumption is that children are naturally inquisitive, explorative, demonstrative, and sensitive. If this is the natural state of a child, then an environment that confines the child in some way is contrary to her fundamental nature. Although children are expected to learn certain rules of social interaction and respect others in their environment, it is not reasonable to expect that most children will thrive in an environment as restrictive as a classroom. Admittedly, there are some schools that respect the individual child and her learning style, providing opportunities for creative discovery and freedom. The majority of schools, however, demand that children conform to more or less rigid expectations for behavior and admonish any significant deviations.

A child may choose one of several styles of reaction to a classroom that suppresses her fundamental nature. Often children learn to repress their natural inclinations and seek styles of behavior that will win them praise and recognition. When a child chooses some other reaction, such as rebellion, or simply cannot repress a natural exuberance for learning and social interaction, then the whole industry of academic disciplinarians, psychologists, and physicians is brought into the game.

The irony is that the industry sees itself as humanizing the treatment of children. Instead of blaming children for their antisocial behavior, this new field seeks to identify a disorder that underlies the symptoms. The identification and labeling of Attention Deficit Disorder (ADD) and ADHD (Attention Deficit Hyperactivity Disorder) provide a mechanism for chemical investigation and chemical treatment. When our children are distracted by the world around them, impulsive in their pursuit of creative ideas, and craving active exploration of the world and their own innate urges, they are given a diagnosis. This restrictive attitude gives a clear message about what we value. The child receives the message that she needs to be fixed. Parents become convinced that something is wrong with their child. Then the child's fundamental way of being in the world is seen as a disease that requires treatment with drugs. The use of these drugs, however, is fraught with problems including many side effects (sleep disturbance, appetite suppression, weight loss, growth delays, nervous tics, loss of creativity, and depression). Drugging children so they can conform in the classroom setting may be thwarting our best intentions for developing innovative, creative thinkers who can solve problems in unusual and distinctive ways. Conformity may be leading our students to mediocrity.

It's much more appropriate for parents to understand their child's attention skills so that a combination of demystification, self-understanding, and natural treatment pave the way to success. The problems created by attention disorders should not be minimized. Children are often demoralized or identified as troublemakers if their distractibility, impulsivity, and restlessness create significant classroom disruptions. Several specific areas of attention dysfunction have been correlated with learning problems. This is not surprising since attention skills are required to accurately perceive, store, and retrieve information. In one study, 73 percent of a group of 422 children with attention dysfunction had evidence of learning problems (Accardo et al., 1990). Other studies have shown an association between the temperament categories describing attention problems (distractibility, low persistence, and high activity) with grades in reading and achievement scores in reading and math (Martin and Holbrook, 1985).

It should also be recognized and acknowledged that creativity and attention "problems" often go hand in hand. The highly creative individual has the ability to take disparate pieces of information and join them in completely new ways. Creative people are often dissatisfied with the mundane and seek excitement. They tend to be enthusiastic, restless, and impulsive—the same traits that get them labeled with ADHD or ADD. Inventors, innovators, entrepreneurs, and artistic geniuses of all sorts have been diagnosed with attention disorder, either during their life or posthumously (Thomas Edison, Ben Franklin, Mozart, Walt Disney). There may be significant value in having ADD or ADHD traits. And there is concern among many researchers that Ritalin and other stimulant medications used to treat symptoms suppress creativity (Armstrong, 1997).

Focus Control, Behavior, and Attentiveness

If parents and educators understand the attention functions of each child, then they can create the best possible learning environment and educational program for that individual child. Attention functions fall into three categories: focus and concentration, behavior or intention, and attentiveness. Many children have strengths in some of these areas and difficulties with aspects of others. In fact, adults and children all have stronger and weaker areas of attention controls. Understanding both strengths and weaknesses in learning functions, including attention, paves the way to the development of strategies for learning more efficiently. If you know that a child is easily distracted by visual cues in the environment, then keep a focused light on her study area at home and dim the lights in the room. If you know that a socially inclined child gets tempted away from her work at school by her friends' distracting conversations, attempt to have her desk situated away from her closest friends. These bypass strategies are simple preventive measures that minimize the effects of attention styles that may interfere with successful work. They do not suppress a child's natural exuberance or creativity.

Focus and concentration involve the ability to stay on track and pay attention. This ability depends upon several important skills. Students need to attend to the salient details, ignoring irrelevant information, such as the extraneous text in a math word problem. Their focal strength allows them to keep the big picture in mind while observing and defining the relevant details that explain why the big picture is true.

Students also need to maintain an inner dialogue, monitoring their own work to make sure they are solving the problem, gathering the right information from their reading, or expressing fluent and cohesive statements in their writing. Expressing ideas and using correct language are simultaneous tasks that require both focus and the feedback responses of self-monitoring.

Several types of control mechanisms are also required for disciplined and successful focus and concentration. Students sometimes need to control their sensory (auditory and visual) distractibility, ignoring attractive sights and sounds that will take them off track. Similarly, they need to resist their inner distractions at times, delaying the gratification of desires that arise while doing less compelling tasks. And finally, they need to delay their verbal communication with friends and classmates until appropriate times for social interaction, since there are constant opportunities in the classroom for social distraction.

All of these skills develop gradually in children. A first-grader is more likely to become distracted while working than a third-grader. If children are taught about these attention functions, then they will have more awareness to develop and practice their self-controls in distracting settings. This type of self-understanding can be invaluable as part of a training program for all school-age children.

Behavior or intention is the second category of attention functions. Children also need to attend to the way they behave or express their inner drives. These intention functions include motor control, the ability to sit still when appropriate, and behavior control. Some children have a tendency to react quickly either in anger with aggressive behaviors or on impulse, blurting out responses in class or disrupting the flow of the classroom by expressing their own personal opinions at inopportune moments. These children tend to be restless and intrusive, often responding without forethought.

ATTENTION AND INTENTION FUNCTIONS

Strength	Weakness
FOCUS AND CONCENTRATION:	
Focal strength and quality	Misses salient details
Self-monitoring and self-correction	Careless mistakes and miscues
Sensory control	Auditory and visual distractibility
Appetite control	Insatiability; distracted by desires
Social control	Distracted by peers
BEHAVIOR OR INTENTION:	
Motor control	Overactive
Behavior control	Disruptive; aggressive
Reflective forethought and planning	Impulsive
ATTENTIVENESS:	
Sleep-arousal balance	Tired and sleepy when studying
Associative control	Daydreaming

The third attention realm is what we might call **attentiveness**. Some children get tired out by thinking, or they get sleepy when listening to instructions or lectures. They may suffer from a problem with sleep-arousal balance arising from a variety of causes. Allergies can cause daytime tiredness. Interrupted breathing during sleep can result in a tired child during the day. An even more common problem is a deficiency of controls over free associations. These children are daydreamers, distracted by their own creative imaginations at times when they need to listen to or watch a demonstration or instructions.

Managing Attention Problems

The first step when addressing attention functions is to understand them in the individual child. Parents who discover and describe their child's attention styles will have a tremendous advantage in developing strategies that improve attention and define when apparent problems may actually be strengths. For example, once parents understand that a child's impulsive style is the very nature of the creative process and that most breakthrough ideas are impulsive, they can achieve a deep appreciation for the exuberance that has previously been so frustrating. This can lead them to develop ways to enhance and enrich their child's experience of her own impulsivity. The cure then lies within the awareness. Then their understanding becomes a spark to develop solutions that can take the form of enrichment, bypass strategies, and advocacy in the school system. When parents see the child's emotional reactions to frustration in their true light, they can take steps to correct the situation rather than continue in their own emotionally charged responses to the child.

This understanding occurs in the child as self-awareness. As soon as a child is told, possibly for the first time, that distractibility is a tremendous advantage, she is freed from her previous negative reinforcement and empowered to achieve a higher level of self-confidence. Distractibility and hyperattentiveness to the environment can lead to constant discovery and personal evolution. Daydreaming can open the doors to dimensions that are hidden behind the mind's limiting control mechanisms. If creativity and intuitive understanding are the keys to reality, a child with free-ranging association is at a distinct advantage for the process of discovery. The problem is that these qualities are usually only admired in accomplished adults who have rejected many of society's values. Our culture is so intent on rationality as the most valuable commodity of mind, and children's creativity is constantly suppressed. Those qualities that foster natural creative expression deserve our recognition. A child who feels this admiration for her true nature will blossom. Then areas of attention that are weak can be addressed. But they must be seen in perspective and the child must feel validated for who she is as a creative being.

The correct homeopathic medicine can free the child. This is especially true in the area of attention. Since attention problems reflect an imbalance in the body, they will usually normalize under the action of a remedy. For example, in a child who cannot remain still long enough to focus on a task, the homeopathic medicine will enhance the natural ability to calm the mind and willfully bring motor activity under control. This is an ability that a homeopathic medicine encourages in the same way that immune system function improves after homeopathic treatment.

Similarly, Chinese medicine views attention problems as an overactive response to an energetic deficiency state. For example, the underlying deficiency of Kidney yin allows Liver yang to become excessive. Stated another way, the lack of controls allows unwanted, random energy to rise up, causing the syndrome of restlessness and impulsivity. The treatment principle in Chinese medicine is to tonify the deficiency while calming the disturbance using stimulation of acupuncture points and herbs.

Dietary interventions that improve attention include eating foods high in phosphatidylserine (eggs), taking a fish oil supplement with vitamin E, and avoiding the food triggers that interfere with concentration and efficient brain function (see page 21).

School Management

The most difficult aspect of attention problems is not understanding the child, but coping with the artificial environment of school. This is because the child is infinitely flexible and schools are structurally rigid. Parents may have significant ability to change the school setting, either by moving the child to a school that is a better fit or by helping the teacher to adjust her style of relating to this child. A supportive, caring, and responsive teacher can often work wonders in a situation that has previously been so frustrating. Suggestions that will make the teacher's life easier are often readily accepted, especially if they are simple and offered in a spirit of cooperation. For example, a child with auditory distractibility will benefit from frequent repetition and reinforcement with written lesson plans and material consistently presented in a visual format. These kinds of bypass strategies that seek to avoid the weakest areas of attention will usually enable children to process more efficiently. Other useful techniques include seating the child closer to the teacher, and developing a code system for the teacher and student to use for communication about attention issues. For example, when the teacher senses that the student's mind seems to be wandering, she can bring her back to the task with a gentle touch on the shoulder. Allowing an active child to learn while moving around the classroom, sending her on frequent errands to the school office, or appointing her to coordinate field trips and other activities will focus the student's energy on tasks that liberate her kinetic energy. There are hundreds of these types of interventions in the literature dedicated to attention problems (see the appendix for recommendations).

These types of communication devices can be established at a meeting with parents, student, and teacher. Many teachers will respond to an open and positive approach to solving these attention issues, although they all have a limit as to how far they are willing to put themselves out for an individual child, especially one who has already managed to consume what seems like inordinate amounts of classroom time. A preventive approach is often useful. Meet with a new teacher at the beginning of the school year and communicate about the best teaching styles that seem to work with this individual student. Teachers usually welcome this proactive approach.

Learning Styles

The most important advice that I can give to parents of children during the early elementary school years is to read with them every day. Reading stories to children will foster a love for the written word. Talking about books you read will promote an inquisitive and thoughtful approach to written material. Encouraging your child to read to you will also allow you to personally assess her progress and determine when she is having difficulties with reading or comprehension. You are the closest person to your child, and you are most qualified to detect possible learning problems. You may not be a professional educator, but you are extremely familiar with your child's successes and frustrations. If you are concerned about a possible learning problem or area of weakness, you can bring it to the attention of teachers and educational specialists to obtain their opinions. Remember, however, that you are the manager of your child's education, and you are responsible for her academic success.

Find the subjects that fascinate your child and pursue them. Go to the library to find books about trains or dinosaurs or doll manufacturing or figure skating or veterinarians—whatever interests your child the most. Encourage your child to become an expert in her area of specialization. Encourage writing in a journal, creating stories, and drawing pictures about these subjects. She can begin writing her own books beginning in first grade and continuing throughout the school years, developing more and more complexity and rigor in her creations. If your child is less inclined to do written work than other forms of expression, then adjust these projects to her own style of learning. If she is more inclined to active learning, then build organized collections. Get books about science projects or natural history exploration and pursue those. Use clay modeling and collages if your child is particularly tactile. The message should be that learning is fun and something that you encourage by your own participation. Go on field trips for enrichment activities. Encourage your child's discovery of the world. Doing this you will discover your child's strengths and weaknesses in learning skills as well as the particular areas of intelligence that resonate most with her talents.

Basic Learning Skills

The basic learning skills can be separated into four areas: memory, sequential processing, simultaneous processing, and motor skills. Parents should observe these basic skill areas as they manifest in learning as well as daily tasks and play. All other academic skills—including reading, mathematics, and writing—depend upon a complex and multifaceted interplay of these four basic learning skills.

Memory is intimately linked with attention. Registration in memory requires that a child acquire information and selectively sift through the data to determine what should be remembered. If selective attention is impaired, then the data will not be perceived in a form that can be stored in memory. Scrambled reception makes for poor acquisition. Selective attention is also dependent on memory. Children must constantly scan data for the salient facts, but choosing which items are relevant requires that past experiences can be recalled to make comparisons and judgments. A deficient memory will impair this selective process. For example, if a child is writing a report, she must remember past reading experiences to integrate new facts and form a coherent, fluent understanding to convey and explain her thoughts and ideas. In fact, all production tasks require memory functions. The selection of accurate and appropriate language, the tasks of writing that include using proper grammar, spelling, and descriptive abilities all depend upon memory and information access. Problems with memory will have an impact on reading, writing, and math.

If you observe that your child has difficulty remembering lists or household jobs, or if your child continually forgets to bring the right books home from school or forgets to turn in assignments, then you may suspect a memory problem. Fortunately, memory is malleable. It improves over time and you can encourage its development. Teaching your child memory enhancement techniques will both compensate for the weakness and develop a stronger memory. You can encourage your child to repeat facts and rewrite spelling words to register them more firmly in memory. Picturing facts in the mind, combining data into related groups, underlining, and summarizing are all potent aids to memory.

Sequential processing involves the ordering of information into a series, such as the letters in a word, the words in a sentence, or the digits in a number. Sequencing is intimately related to a temporal order—telling time and counting. Sequences form the basis for many early childhood learning tasks including spelling and decoding, time relationships (before and after), reading clocks, arithmetic, and following directions. Tasks in later childhood and adolescence place increasingly complex demands upon sequential processing. Older children are expected to create outlines, appreciate long causal chains of reasoning, and organize their time to work efficiently.

Children with sequencing problems may have a history of difficulty learning to read or telling time. Decoding new or unfamiliar words is especially taxing. Spelling skills are typically poor and organization is often disastrous. If you suspect sequencing problems are interfering with your child's ability to read or write coherent ideas, then you need to discuss it with your child's teacher. Various remedial techniques can improve sequencing skills and an educational specialist can help to solve the problem through appropriate tutoring.

Simultaneous processing involves the understanding or meaning in a complex pattern or configuration. This requires an awareness of pattern formations and the ability to discriminate these patterns from background information and other similar sets of data. This awareness usually occurs through visual processing of spatial configurations. It is therefore often referred to as **visual-spatial** processing. However, auditory information will often contain a similar level of complexity and require the simultaneous processing of a great deal of information. Children may have the ability to appreciate visual-spatial stimuli when they are relatively simple (as in symbol recognition), but they experience difficulty when they are required to complete a more complex simultaneous task. For example, a child may easily decode a word or comprehend a written sentence, but then become overwhelmed reading an information-laden paragraph that calls upon more complex processing skills.

Common problems that parents may notice include letter reversals, trouble identifying specific symbols (letters and numbers), or difficulty learning the sounds and meanings of written words. These children tend to have problems establishing a strong sight vocabulary, or difficulty with motor tasks that involve spatial awareness (drawing or catching a ball).

Motor skills are primarily responsible for output and production. Output problems refer to the child's difficulty encoding information that has been stored and generating a product. This production takes the form of fine motor activity (writing), gross motor activity (running and playing ball), and expressive language. Output problems may manifest as speech problems or a delay in verbal expression. Parents need to be aware though that children develop language at much different rates. Some children simply wait to talk until they are older than the typical 2-year-old who begins to string words together to form ideas and sentences. If children are having problems with enunciation or expressive language as they enter school, a referral to a speech and language therapist may be warranted. There is little evidence, however, that intervention for language delays in a preschooler has a significant effect as long as hearing is adequate. If a parent suspects a hearing problem, then the cause should be determined by a medical professional.

Fine motor problems are often not identified until later elementary school. During the early elementary school years, most academic tasks involve decoding, memory, and passive learning. Tasks such as early reading and arithmetic do not stress output skills. As children proceed into upper grades, more importance is placed on output tasks—handwriting, report writing, and spelling. A problem with motor skills will slow the production process as ideas flow faster than the pencil can record them. These children will benefit from an educational evaluation of these skills because therapy is effective at improving motor function and dexterity.

Learning Styles at School

The ideal academic setting in school includes a program of active learning, an integrated curriculum across subject areas, opportunities for artistic pursuits, music training, and adequate exercise, with teachers trained in the assessment of individual learning styles. Some schools have already achieved this ideal, others are pursuing specific aspects of these goals.

Active learning involves a hands-on approach to education with the use of project-oriented exploration in early education and self-directed research in upper grades. The principle of active learning includes the direct involvement by students in experimentation, discovery, and a self-directed approach to subjects, rather than the passive learning that characterizes a didactic, lecture-based curriculum. Students generally are more stimulated by doing projects that involve probing with questions and researching ideas in several forms like personal interviews, Internet searches, consulting with mentors, and personal discovery.

An integrated curriculum means that students are studying the same topic at the same time in different subject areas, so that history, English, science, art, and sometimes even math are each examining various aspects of a topic. For example, if the topic is Ancient Greece, then the history and culture are also explored through the literature of the era, scientific progress and experimentation of the time are examined, and artistic expression in its various forms portrays the spirit of the Greeks. This immersion in Greek culture demonstrates the interplay of each subject area and provides for a rich and diverse experience with plenty of opportunity to delve deeply into the meaning, philosophy, importance, and relevance of the Greeks to our own culture today.

Many schools are training teachers to identify individual learning styles of their students. A teacher's job can become significantly easier if she gives students learning materials in a form they can most easily process. For students with highly developed simultaneous and visual-spatial processing, she can have them build models and construct diagrams. For students with more affinity for linear, text-based learning, she can emphasize more research reports, writing tasks, and debates. There are national programs for this type of teacher training available through the All Kinds of Minds Institute (www.allkindsofminds.org). Their program Schools Attuned trains the entire teaching staff of a school.

Children can also be taught how their own minds work. This self-understanding can do wonders to enable students to bypass their weak areas of learning skills. It can also help them identify their strengths and develop pride in their abilities. If a child knows what she does well, then she will probably use this strength to its maximum advantage, building expertise and accomplishment that in turn foster high self-esteem. Children who use their strongest learning skills to overcome weaker areas will have more success. Whether their strengths lie in the areas of memory, visual processing, or auditory skills, understanding them and then discovering ways to rely upon them will make any child's educational experience that much easier and rewarding. Renowned pediatrician Mel Levine has written two books directed to children for this purpose and several for parents as well (see the appendix).

Electronics: Television, Video Games, and Cell Phones
Television

An overwhelming body of medical literature has documented the negative effects of television viewing on children. More than 1,000 studies have shown an association between aggressive and violent behaviors in children and their exposure to violent television programming (Strasburger, 2002). Television also promotes obesity (Marshall et al., 2004), contributes to attention problems (Christakis, 2004), interferes with academic performance (Strasburger, 1986), and encourages the initiation of sexual behavior (Collins et al., 2004).

Given the significant problems that television exposure can create in children, and the questionable role-modeling and consumer choices that television encourages, it seems wise for parents to limit their children's time spent in front of the screen. Parents can control what programming their children watch as well as the amount of time they spend. Educational videos and movies with a more positive message and less gratuitous violence represent a far better choice for children than most cartoons. Commercial advertising stimulates a calculated consumerism in children, purposefully seeking to manipulate their tastes and develop a nagging factor to undermine parental authority (Linn, 2004).

Limiting television exposure seems warranted in all situations. Delay the onset of television exposure as long as possible. It seems reasonable that television viewing at an early age will cause more learning problems than at a later age. If your children do watch television, limit the number of hours. The U.S. Department of Education estimates that children watch an average of three to five hours of television every day. These children will view 12,000 acts of violence every year. Most television shows for children contain twenty violent acts per hour. One or two hours a day is the maximum children should spend in front of the television. Many families have a no-television rule during the week.

Parents need to enforce age-appropriate rules for programs their children may watch. There are many television shows that encourage learning and socially appropriate behaviors for preschool-age children. Some cartoons have a minimum amount of violence and a generally positive message. The TV Parental Guidelines Monitoring Board has established a rating system by age group for television shows. The TVY rating signifies programming designed for children age 2 to 6. The TVG rating signifies programming deemed suitable for all ages by the Parental Guidelines Board. All other rating categories include programs with violent acts, coarse language, or sexual situations. Every television manufactured after the year 2000 contains the V-chip that displays the Parental Guidelines ratings for children's television content. You can activate the V-chip on your TV by consulting the menu or your owner's manual. The V-chip can block programming by age-based category or content label. When you block a particular rating or content label, all categories beyond that will be blocked.

Be aware of the content of shows your children watch. Sit down and view these programs with your child. Discuss them. Discuss the commercials, or mute the commercials. Better yet: Read a book with your child, explore a garden, dig in a sandbox, visit a museum, go to the local zoo or aquarium, visit a pet store, assign a research project, or encourage your child's interest in a hobby. If you are one of the brave parents who dares to turn off the television, good for you.

Video Games

The violence of television programming is multiplied exponentially in video games because violent acts that a child perpetrates are encouraged and rewarded. Killing is portrayed as a benign act with no negative consequences, and players must become more violent to win. Violent video games are associated with aggressive behaviors and delinquency (Anderson and Dill, 2000).

Video games, like television programs and movies, have a rating system: EC for Early Childhood 3+, E for Everyone 6+, T for Teen 13+ (guaranteed to contain violence), M for Mature, and A for Adult. Parents would be well advised to note the ratings and watch while their children play these games. Certainly the amount of time spent with video games (or computer games) needs to be limited so that the game playing does not interfere with time available for studies, reading, and other more creative pursuits. Video games have an addicting quality that eats up inordinate amounts of time. Teens especially can get hooked on the challenges and ascending levels of a particular video game or online game with its own blend of fascination, community of players, and particular form of culture.

Cell Phones

The medical literature unequivocally suggests that cell phones are associated with an increased risk of brain tumors. Enough studies have shown this connection to warrant caution in cell phone use, particularly with children. The antenna of a cell phone emits significant amounts of electromagnetic radiation that penetrates the skull. The penetration is greater in children than in adults. One study at the Spanish Neuro Diagnostic Research Institute examined the brain wave activity of an 11-year-old boy and a 13-year-old girl during cell phone use. The researchers found that brain waves were significantly altered and remained abnormal for up to an hour after the call. They suggested that this alteration in brain waves could be associated with memory loss, poor concentration, and aggressive behavior (Hyland, 2000). Cell phones have also been linked to immune system dysfunction, headaches, dizziness, depression, cellular aging, and Alzheimer's disease.

A review of all cell phone studies to date revealed that nine published studies have examined the association between cell phones and brain or eye tumors. All nine showed an enhanced cancer risk from cell phones with increasing risk for longer duration of phone use (Kundi et al., 2004).

In the year 2000, less than 20 percent of American teens owned a cell phone. By 2004, more than half of all teens owned one. Given the amount of time that teenagers spend on the phone, the potential for health problems is alarming.

The basic principles of child safety require that we eliminate cell phone dangers and the potential for bodily harm that they pose. Children should not put cell phones next to their bodies or heads. Cell phones emit radiation whether they are in talk or standby mode as they constantly search for a transmitter. If children use a cell phone, they should always use a headset. This should be a rule as strictly enforced as use of a seatbelt. Cell phones should be kept in a backpack or purse, not in a pocket near the reproductive organs.

PART THREE

MANAGING ACUTE ILLNESS

CHAPTER 10

Home Treatment

The Role of Natural Treatment

The goal of this part of the book is to support your child through acute illnesses safely, without compromising his health with drug treatment. Acute illnesses are defined as self-limited sets of symptoms that are not recurrent or part of an underlying chronic condition such as asthma or allergy. Infectious illnesses are usually acute (chicken pox, colds, stomach flu). Other symptoms such as hives and diarrhea, or the discomforts of teething, are common acute situations that are also amenable to natural treatment.

By "natural treatment" I mean those forms of support that stimulate immune function, strengthen the body's ability to react in a positive way to illness, and provide the tools for recovery. Pharmaceutical drugs do none of these things, so their use should be limited. There is nothing wrong with using drugs when necessary, but a holistic pediatric approach to illness seldom requires them. Drugs will sometimes provide relief from suffering, so there is some use for painkillers. Antibiotics may give the body a rest from fighting bacteria so that other forms of treatment can stimulate recovery. However, most conventional medications given in acute situations such as colds, coughs, ear infections, digestive upset, and fevers are ineffective and interfere with healing.

When to Treat Illness at Home

Parents are the perfect first providers of care for acute illness. Armed with a little knowledge, a kit of supplies, and a telephone for back-up, you are ready to treat most of your child's symptoms and illnesses without any medical training or need for other medical providers. You are the first ones on the scene, and you can provide the first forms of care. In most situations this is all that is needed.

Your calm reassurance, affection, touch, holding, and attention will do wonders to decrease symptoms. Most children are easily upset; their emotions surface quickly and readily, and acute symptoms can be distressing for them. Injuries, pain, and unusual changes in bodily function can be frightening for children. Providing comfort to them and pronouncing the time-honored phrases of reassurance—"You're OK" and "It will go away soon"—will calm these fears and the accompanying symptoms. You learned during prenatal classes about the "fear, tension, pain" cycle. Applying this approach to children will relieve their anxiety, stress hormones, and pain responses. Relaxation relieves stress and tension, and will stimulate healing.

Safety and Common Sense

Acute illness is usually benign, not dangerous to children, and will resolve on its own, especially with a little help in the right direction. If you are alarmed at your child's symptoms, then that is always the time to seek help from a medical provider. The following chapter of this book, and other health guides listed in the recommended books section of the Appendix, provide guidelines about when to seek additional care for your child. Safety should always be your primary concern. Ninety percent of childhood symptoms go away readily with a little supportive care. Another small percentage will benefit from the care of an experienced holistic provider. It is rare that you will need an emergency room, urgent care facility, or high-tech medical interventions. However, situations do happen when urgent care is needed. Appendicitis, pneumonia, meningitis, and cellulitis, for example, are serious childhood acute illnesses that require careful medical management. None of these can be handled at home.

Here are some general rules regarding home care of illness. If your child seems very sick, lethargic, or listless, seek medical advice. If an unusual symptom occurs that you cannot easily explain, call your provider. If your child is having difficulty breathing, call immediately. If your child is not recovering in an appropriate time frame based on the information you know about a disease process, ask a professional's opinion.

Naturally, you will be more inclined to call a holistic provider if you have one available, because his or her advice will be more in tune with your own philosophy of health care, and he or she is likely to offer advice that you can implement. An allopathic doctor is more likely to suggest drugs at an earlier stage of an illness, and you may be more reluctant to call or take your child to the doctor knowing that treatment is likely to be ineffective or contrary to your own preferences. Nonetheless, it is often essential that a child receive a diagnosis for the sake of safety. The sections in Chapter 11 should help you to make decisions about the need to seek professional care.

Home Prescribing

Chapter 11 discusses acute illness and symptoms. It does not cover any chronic illness patterns or the acute, episodic flare-ups of chronic conditions (asthma, eczema, reflux). I have included only those treatments that I know are effective. In my experience homeopathy is the easiest and most effective form of treatment for children's acute illnesses. Kids love the taste of homeopathic medicines, they respond quickly, and they never suffer any side effects. Other forms of treatment can be useful as well, and these are interspersed in the text wherever appropriate. I have simplified the prescribing choices for you because other homeopathic reference books are often difficult for parents to use. Accurate homeopathic prescribing for acute illness depends on an ability to differentiate between medicines using subtleties of symptoms and aggravating influences on symptoms as our guide. This is a difficult process in children's cases because of their relative inability to observe and describe symptoms. Homeopathic clinicians rely to a great extent on their experience and familiarity with children's illnesses and the effectiveness of particular medicines. I have translated my own experience into the choices I provide for you in each section.

Here are some suggestions for the use of homeopathic medicines. The choice of the medicine is important. Give only one homeopathic medicine at a time. It is possible for one medicine to interfere with the action of another and send mixed and confusing messages to the body. The medicine's strength or potency, the dosage, and the frequency of repetition are of negligible importance. Any strength is likely to work (from a 6X potency to a 200C). The strength is determined by the number of times the medicine has been subjected to the homeopathic pharmaceutical process. The C or centesimal range of potencies is stronger than the X or decimal range, and a higher number indicates a stronger or more deep-acting form of the medicine. I generally recommend that parents use 30C medicines, but that choice is rather arbitrary; a 6X or 12C is likely to work just as well. Similarly, the dosage is unimportant. A homeopathic medicine will work if you give one pellet or five. There is absolutely no toxicity involved, and a child can safely eat the contents of an entire bottle of homeopathic medicine with no untoward effects. One dose of a medicine is just as likely to work as taking it three times per day or every two hours. In general, once a homeopathic medicine is acting beneficially, it is wise to stop and not continue repetitions. On the other hand, children tend to burn off the effect of a homeopathic medicine during an illness, and I usually recommend repeating the medicine until symptoms are clearly improved. The stronger the force of the illness, the more repetitions are appropriate. For a normal cold or cough, three doses per day is usually adequate given the proviso that once symptoms clearly improve it is wise to stop and wait. Repeating the medicine later if symptoms return is always an option.

Homeopathic medicines are equally and completely safe for newborns, infants, and older children. Dosage is typically one or two pellets of sugar pills that have been prepared by a homeopathic pharmacy. Infants can hold the pellets in their cheeks and they will dissolve. Older children can chew them.

If a medicine is not working, then consider either consulting a more detailed homeopathic home prescribing book to find a medicine more closely aligned with the presenting symptoms, or consult with a homeopathic professional.

I do not recommend over-the-counter combination homeopathic remedies. I do not typically find them as effective as the well-chosen single medicine. The theory behind these combinations is the shotgun approach: Throw several typically indicated medicines at a symptom and see if one is correct. I am concerned that giving several incorrect homeopathic medicines confuses the body's reactions and can upset the delicate equilibrium and balance of a child's system.

Homeopathic medicines are readily available in health food stores and in various home-prescribing kits made by the homeopathic pharmacies. I have referred to all homeopathic medicines using italics to distinguish them from other products. In the following sections I also recommend herbs and some pediatric herbal formulas that are only available from practitioners. In that case you may want your medical provider to order herbal formulas for you to keep at home. See the Appendix.

Both Western and Chinese herbal prescriptions are best administered in liquid extracts. I recommend continuing herbs until the symptoms are gone.

Each section also contains suggestions for acupuncture massage (acupressure or *tui na*). These massage points will stimulate healing and relieve symptoms. Repeat each suggestion 50–100 times at a session while holding your child, or while your child is sleeping. The gentle massage is soothing and reassuring to your child during times of illness.

CHAPTER 11

Treating Common Symptoms

Introduction

For detailed instructions about the proper use of homeopathic medicines and the general approach to home treatment of ailments, see Chapter 10. This chapter outlines the steps to take in evaluating and treating acute illnesses and symptoms in your child. The sections are arranged in alphabetical order. Each section also contains a list of warning signs that should lead you to consult a medical provider. The illness patterns described in this chapter apply to acute or short-term and self-limited problems, not to chronic long-term and recurring patterns of symptoms. Chronic illnesses such as asthma, eczema, and weakened immune function will require the help of a holistic health care provider.

Abdominal Pain

Symptoms

For practical purposes, abdominal pain can be separated into several types: infant colic, stomach aches, and lower abdominal pain. Colic is discussed in its own section (see page 225). For older children, stomach aches are common, and usually easily treated. Toddlers, preschoolers, and even 5–6-year-olds may identify any number of normal sensations as stomach aches, including hunger, gas, and the need to have a bowel movement. Other stomach and intestinal ailments can be viral, including those illnesses with vomiting and diarrhea that tend to go around the family (see page 230). Constipation is also a trigger of abdominal pain. If you suspect that your child is in pain from constipation, see your medical provider. Do not attempt home treatment.

Recurrent episodes of abdominal pain or stomach aches have many causes including emotional reactions, chronic constipation, parasites, deficient spleen *chi*, food allergies, systemic yeast infection, and many others. These are not acute problems and should be treated by a qualified medical provider.

Treatment

The two most commonly indicated homeopathic medicines for stomach aches are *Arsenicum album* and *Nux vomica*.

Arsenicum is most often indicated when pain or vomiting begins in the middle of the night. If a child has been exposed to someone with stomach flu and symptoms begin suddenly with vomiting, then *Arsenicum* is usually the first choice. Children who need *Arsenicum* may also be chilly, lethargic, or anxious.

Nux vomica can be used if you suspect food is involved. If your child has eaten something you suspect may have caused symptoms, or if she has overeaten and gets a stomach ache, for example after a birthday party, then *Nux vomica* is the remedy to choose. *Nux vomica* symptoms may also include nausea and vomiting. If diarrhea is present, then *Arsenicum* is usually more appropriate.

Abdominal pain can be very crampy, with children bending double and crying. In this instance, the first medicine to consider is *Colocynth*. If that relieves the symptoms quickly, then you can be assured it is an intestinal cramp or gas. If it recurs in this intense form, or if it persists, consult your medical provider. Several potentially dangerous conditions

---

DANGER SIGNS WITH ABDOMINAL PAIN

If abdominal pain lasts more than an hour, call your child's medical provider.

Before calling for advice, take your child's temperature.

If abdominal pain is severe, seek medical attention.

If abdominal pain persists despite homeopathic treatment, seek help through your provider or an urgent care facility.

---

manifest as abdominal pain, often accompanied by vomiting. These include appendicitis, intussesception (acute obstruction of the intestines), and other types of infections. Appendicitis can be diagnosed with a physical exam, ultrasound, and blood test. The danger of appendicitis is a burst appendix and generalized infection through the abdominal cavity.

Give only sips of water if your child has been vomiting. Sucking on ice chips works well because it is difficult to get too much at a time. When your child resumes eating after the stomach flu, begin with mild foods that are easy to digest (plain yogurt, applesauce, soups) before proceeding to more challenging foods.

Apply a hot water bottle or heating pad to relieve cramping.

Acupressure Massage

Press on the points Stomach 36, Stomach 41, and Spleen 6 on the lower leg and ankle. Stomach 36 is located about an inch below the knee just to the outside of the shinbone. Stomach 41 is located on the front of the ankle, at the midline. Spleen 6 is located about an inch above the prominent bone on the inside of the ankle. On older children, the distance is a little more. Find the tender spot and press on it.

Lightly rub the abdomen in a full circle, first in a clockwise direction thirty-six times, then in a counter-clockwise direction thirty-six times.

Bites and Stings

Symptoms

Insect bites cause annoying, itching hives around the site of the bite, but stings from bees and wasps tend to cause more dramatic swelling and discomfort, and they can result in dangerous allergic reactions. An allergic reaction consists of difficulty breathing and a feeling that the throat is swelling. Seek immediate medical attention for suspected allergic reactions to stings. A swollen area around the site of a bite or sting represents a local reaction, not an allergic reaction, even if it covers quite an extensive area.

Tick and spider bites should not usually cause any significant problems. However, a small percentage of one species of tick may infect humans with a bacterium that causes Lyme disease. The symptoms of Lyme disease include a rash in the shape of a ring around the site of the bite; the rash appears seven to fourteen days after the bite, and is followed in a few days by flu symptoms and joint or muscle pain. If any of these symptoms occur after a tick bite, see your medical provider. Most spider bites are harmless, except those of the black widow and brown recluse spiders. Black widow bites will cause sweating, stomach cramps, nausea, headache, and dizziness. Brown recluse spider bites result in a bull's-eye marking, a blister surrounded by white and red circles, and flu-like symptoms. Both of these spider bites are extremely dangerous to children and require immediate emergency care.

DANGER SIGNS WITH BITES

If your child is suffering with wheezing, difficult breathing, or throat swelling as a result of a sting, seek immediate medical care.

A black widow or recluse spider bite should be treated immediately at an emergency room.

Treatment

Itchy bites from mosquitoes, fleas, and chiggers, as well as painful bites from spiders and stings from bees and wasps, respond very well to a dose or two of *Ledum palustre*. An excellent gel that relieves itching also contains *Ledum* along with Echinacea and Urtica dioica (SSSSting Stop, by Boericke & Tafel). Applying Aloe vera gel or Echinacea can also be effective. Apply ice or a cold compress to bites and stings to stop the spread of the histamine that results in itching and swelling.

If a child is stung by a bee or wasp, check to see if the stinger is still imbedded in the skin. If you see it, scrape it out with your fingernail. Do not grasp it and pull it. That will cause more venom from the venom sac to be injected into the skin, worsening the reaction.

If you know or suspect that your child has an allergic reaction to stings, consult your medical provider about getting a prescription for an epinephrine kit that provides you with the means to prevent life-threatening symptoms.

If you find a tick attached to your child's skin, remove it with tweezers. Grasp the tick near the skin and gently pull until the tick releases its hold. Do not twist the tick, do not grasp it with your fingers, and do not attempt to kill it first prior to removal. Watch your child for the onset of the typical rash and illness in seven to fourteen days.

Chicken Pox

Chicken pox is typically a mild and benign disease of childhood. Complications are rare and usually mild. The disease is caused by the varicella-zoster virus, a member of the herpes virus family.

Symptoms

Chicken pox usually begins with a fever and runny nose within eleven to nineteen days after exposure. Some children have no symptoms prior to the appearance of the typical eruptions. These are small, flat, pink areas that soon develop a clear fluid-filled center, and then open and crust over within two to three days. They appear in crops, and persist as active lesions for a week. During this time children are contagious and usually uncomfortable and itchy, especially if they have many eruptions or if these occur on mucous membranes. The disease usually ends uneventfully after a week, and children then have permanent immunity to future exposure. When all lesions are crusted over (usually by day seven), your child is no longer contagious.

Treatment

Treatment is directed at making children comfortable. Homeopathic treatment may be helpful for the itching and other bothersome symptoms. Usually the only medicine needed is *Rhus tox* when itching is bothersome. If the illness is characterized by a high fever, see the Fevers section (see page 235). If eruptions are becoming inflamed, infected, or full of pus, then give *Antimonium crudum*.

Two home remedies are useful for itching. Oatmeal powder (the Aveeno brand packages, available at most drugstores) work well, added to a tub. Calamine lotion applied to the individual itchy lesions will relieve symptoms. Do not use calamine that contains camphor because of the risk of antidoting homeopathic medicines.

I do not recommend giving fever reducers for chicken pox symptoms. Aspirin should never be used during chicken pox because of the danger of causing Reye's syndrome, which can result in brain damage or death. Allopathic antiviral drugs (acyclovir) have only minimal effect on reducing symptoms or the duration of illness. Risking side effects of any allopathic drug in the treatment of this benign illness is unwarranted.

Colds

Symptoms

Usually a cold begins with a runny nose and tiredness. Sometimes babies are just fussy. These symptoms may be accompanied by fever or sore throat (see those sections in this chapter). Allergies do not cause fevers. Neither does teething, though colds often accompany teething, probably because the stress and pain of getting teeth may lower resistance. Exposure to cold or wet weather may also lower resistance. Viruses cause colds, and they are spread easily from one child to another. If it's going around, it's probably a cold. If it's not accompanied by a change in energy or fussiness, it may be allergies.

Time to Recovery

Often a child's body will fight off a cold in a few days without any treatment, but using natural remedies will promote healing and help prevent complications. Typical colds last for seven days, though congestion may persist longer. Colds are usually contagious for the first three to four days. Keep your child at home at the beginning of colds and for twenty-four hours after fevers have abated.

Sometimes a cold will worsen and progress to include deep coughs or a thick green nasal discharge. These are possible signs of complicating infections, which may be bacterial.

DANGER SIGNS WITH COLDS

See a medical provider if any of the following symptoms are present:

Persistent high fever of 102–103°F

Severe sore throat

Loose, rattling cough or wheezing (high-pitched breathing)

Ear pain, or tugging on the ears in babies

Any fever in a baby less than three months old

Prolonged illness, significant lethargy with unresponsiveness, or severe pain

---

Treatment

The goal of treatment is to give a boost to the immune system so that it fights off the infection efficiently. This can be done with herbs and homeopathic medicines. Both can be given at the same time.

Echinacea: Non-alcoholic, glycerin preparations of the herb Echinacea are prepared specifically for children. Some of them also contain vitamin C. Mix the Echinacea with juice or water. Most health food stores stock Echinacea preparations. Avoid products that contain other herbs or fillers. Golden seal is not needed for colds. Echinacea stimulates the body to produce more white blood cells that fight invasion by viruses or bacteria. Echinacea is not appropriate for allergic symptoms, and should not be used over an extended period of time. Stop when the cold symptoms improve, or after five days.

Directions: Mix with juice or give it straight.

Dosage: For babies under 1 year, 10 drops three times per day; for children over 1 year, 20 drops three times per day.

Windbreaker: This is a Chinese herbal formula designed for children (Chinese Modular Solutions). Yin Chao Junior is a comparable formula (Health Concerns). It stimulates a healing reaction in the body, dispels invasion of cold, and relieves mucus production and congestion. Use it at the onset of colds and continue as long as congestion persists. Shake the bottle before each use. This formula contains alcohol.

Directions: Mix the drops in a small amount of steaming hot water to evaporate the alcohol, then mix this solution with juice.

Dosage: For babies under 1 year, 10 drops three times per day; for children over 1 year, 20 drops three times per day; for children age 3 or older, 3 droppers three times per day.

Vitamin C

Give babies 500 mg vitamin C in powder form, children 1–3 years old 1,000 mg in powder or liquid, and children age 3 or older 2,000 mg per day in divided doses. Use either a powdered form of vitamin C (a buffered preparation such as calcium ascorbate works well in juice or a smoothie) or vitamin C drops. Do not use chewable vitamin C. The acid in contact with molars can cause tooth decay.

Homeopathic Medicines

For stage 1 of the cold, *Allium cepa* is the first remedy to give for a clear runny nose. Or give *Belladonna* if there is also a fever with a clear runny nose. Once the discharge has changed from clear to yellow or green, these remedies are no longer indicated.

For stage 2 of the cold, give *Pulsatilla* when there is a thicker nasal discharge and clingy behavior.

For stage 3 of the cold, *Kali bichromicum* will relieve a thick, green, persisting nasal discharge.

Supportive Measures

If a baby has difficulty nursing because of nasal obstruction, or an older child has trouble sleeping, take her into the bathroom and steam it up with the hot shower. Let her breathe the steam for five minutes. This will loosen things up. Humidifiers and vaporizers are inefficient, messy, and tend to produce and distribute mold.

Acupressure Massage

Repeat each maneuver 100 or more times.

For the first stages of a cold (with clear nasal discharge):

Massage the ring finger on the palm side from the tip to the base in one direction only.

Massage along a line on the lateral side of the forearm (the thumb side) from the wrist to the elbow in one direction only.

Press on a point in the soft web of the thumb and index finger, squeezing with your thumb and index fingers on the front and back of your child's hand.

For the later stages of a cold (with thick green discharge):

Massage the ring finger on the palm side from the base to the tip in one direction only.

Massage along a line in the center of the inside of the forearm from the wrist to the elbow in one direction only.

If accompanied by sinus headache, massage the temples and press on the point at the soft junction of the thumb and index finger.

Colic

Infants who cry—that is basically the definition of colic. Videotapes of babies show that most of them cry for a total of two hours per day when all of their fussy spells in a twenty-four-hour period are added together. Anything more than that is defined as colic, which manifests in various degrees of severity.

Chinese medicine interprets colic as a poorly developed spleen/stomach energy system that is easily stressed by the rigors of digesting food, resulting in stagnation in the intestines and accumulation of gas. However, when infants with colic are compared to other babies they do not have more gas on x-rays or any difference in the tissues of their intestines on biopsies.

Symptoms

Crying can be periodic, occurring primarily in the evening, or it can persist and drive parents crazy. Colic can last for a day or two, or go on for months and months. Typically, it miraculously disappears by the third month. Colic ranges in intensity from its mild form, a fussy baby who quiets on being walked and bounced, to its most intense aspect, an inconsolable screamer who drives his sleep-deprived parents to desperation. Colic is often a chronic, constitutional state requiring precise prescribing by an experienced practitioner to afford a cure.

The acute symptoms of colic typically involve tightening the abdomen, passing gas, pulling in the legs, and lusty crying. It is important to observe infants for other signs of problems if they have persistent crying. Vomiting of significant amounts of milk is a possible sign of intestinal obstruction or reflux, where stomach contents pass back up into the esophagus. Reflux is a common, chronic problem in infants

---

Danger Signs with Colic

See a medical provider if any of the following symptoms are present:

Crying with accompanying fever in a baby during the first three months

Persistent crying over several days

Vomiting or frequent spitting-up

---

and requires appropriate treatment by a trained professional. There are excellent natural treatments for persistent colic and for reflux.

Treatment

Acute periodic episodes of colicky symptoms are often due to gas and cramping abdominal pain. The homeopathic medicine most often indicated on an acute level is *Colocynth*, especially if your baby seems better when you press on her abdomen. *Jalapa* is a colic medicine for babies who cry all night and sleep during the day. *Lycopodium* is used primarily when the gas symptoms are prominent and when the late afternoon and evening (4 to 8 PM) are your baby's worst time of day. *Nux vomica* corresponds to an exceedingly irritable baby who is worse in the mornings. These medicines can be administered on an as-needed basis. However, if symptoms persist or continually recur, then a deeper constitutional treatment is needed to solve the underlying imbalance or weakness. Constitutional homeopathic prescribing, Chinese medicine, chiropractic, and osteopathic manipulation can all result in dramatic improvement in symptoms.

An excellent treatment to build digestive function and encourage normal development of the digestive tract is the pediatric Chinese herbal formula Grow and Thrive, made by Chinese Modular Solutions and available through your health care professional.

Other forms of support and interventions for colic are discussed on page 140.

Acupressure massage treatment is the same as that for abdominal pain (see page 217).

Coughs

Coughs are tricky because they come in so many different types with different causes. A little mucus and irritation in the throat will cause coughs with colds. Infection in the larynx may cause croup. Infection in the large airways with mucus production and inflammation will produce a deep, loose cough characterizing bronchitis. A deeper infection with spasms of coughing and a persistent fever may signal pneumonia. Whooping cough, asthmatic coughs, and persistent, chronic coughing from allergies round out the cough spectrum.

The only coughs that parents should be treating at home are those that accompany colds and croupy symptoms that come in the night.

Treatment

Coughs with colds: Here are my three favorite homeopathic cough medicines for kids:

Bryonia for dry coughs with thirst, when the cough is worse from motion

Kali bichromicum for coughs caused by post-nasal drainage into the throat, with thick green nasal discharge or expectoration from the throat

Rumex crispus for paroxysms of coughing that are difficult to stop and worse from lying down, cold air, deep breathing, and laughing

My experience with homeopathic combination cough syrups and most herbal syrups is poor. I do not usually find them effective. It is much more effective to find the correct homeopathic medicine. Chinese herbal cough syrups containing fritillary, perilla, and loquat also work well. The herbal extract Chest Relief, by Chinese Modular Solutions, is also an excellent formula for coughs.

Croupy coughs: Croup is characterized by an unmistakable barking cough like a seal. It often begins suddenly in the night and is accompanied by difficulty breathing and fear. It is commonly preceded by several days of viral cold symptoms—runny nose and fever. There are two immediate interventions for croup. First, take your child into the bathroom and run a hot shower to steam up the room. Sit with your child in your lap, allowing her to breathe the steam. This will usually calm down the symptoms. Second, give the homeopathic medicine *Aconitum*. Paradoxically, cold air may also relieve the symptoms. Parents sometimes find that a frightening case of croup will dissipate in severity on the way to the emergency room; this is due to the colder night air. *Aconitum* is only indicated for that sudden onset of symptoms. The remedy can be repeated every ten or fifteen minutes if necessary. If your child is having significant difficulty breathing, then seek urgent medical care. For a mild barking cough that persists the next day, the indicated medicine is usually *Hepar sulphur*.

Most other coughs are beyond the realm of home prescribing. Attempting to treat allergic coughs, asthma, or whooping cough at home will usually end in frustration and failure. This is the realm for trained and experienced practitioners.

DANGER SIGNS WITH COUGHS

See a medical provider if any of the following symptoms are present:

Wheezing or difficulty breathing

Persistent coughing with weakness

Persistent coughing with fever

Acupressure Massage

Acupressure can help children get relief from coughs:

Rub the line on the lateral anterior surface of the forearm (thumb side) from the wrist to the elbow in one direction only.

Massage a point on the center of the chest between the nipples.

Massage the points on both sides of the back midway between the spine and the edge of the shoulder blade.

A Note about Allopathic Cough Syrups

A study published in the journal *Pediatrics* proves that cough syrups have no effect on children's coughs, their sleep, or the quality of parents' sleep. One of the ingredients of typical cough syrups, dextromethorphan (DM), caused insomnia, and the other ingredient, dyphenhydramine (DPH), caused drowsiness, in the children enrolled in this study. Other studies have shown similar results.

Although these drugs can be purchased over-the-counter, they are not benign. According to citations in the *Pediatrics* report, DM can cause dependence, psychosis, mania, hallucinations, diabetes, and death, while DPH can cause dependence, nervousness, psychosis, seizures, and death (Paul et al., 2004).

Diarrhea

Diarrhea is characterized by frequent loose or watery stools. A child who experiences a few loose stools without other symptoms probably does not need treatment. Intestinal viruses typically start with stomach aches and vomiting, and then proceed to diarrhea. Other causes of diarrhea include a change in diet and water source, unwise selections in eating, and a handful of serious diseases.

The primary danger with diarrhea is dehydration, which occurs when a child is not taking in enough fluids to compensate for the fluid loss. The essential sign of dehydration is weight loss. If your baby or child is not losing weight, then dehydration is unlikely. A 5 percent loss in weight signifies moderate dehydration. A 10 percent loss in weight suggests serious dehydration and the need to seek medical attention immediately. Dehydration can result in an inability to maintain adequate blood pressure, resulting in shock. Babies with diarrhea need to be carefully monitored for signs of dehydration.

Diarrhea can be annoyingly persistent with normal and loose stools that alternate on and off. Fruit juice, raw fruit, and milk are likely to aggravate diarrhea. Applesauce, yogurt, and cooked foods are easier to digest than raw foods and wheat-containing foods. Bananas tend to be binding, and maintenance of a normal diet is appropriate after the immediate symptoms of an intestinal virus have abated. Diarrhea persisting for more than a few days should be treated by your natural medicine practitioner.

Treatment

Home treatment for diarrhea consists of giving a probiotic intestinal bacteria supplement (*acidophilus* and *bifidus*), a homeopathic medicine, and an additional electroyte solution (either Pedialyte or a homemade rehy-

SIGNS OF DEHYDRATION

Weight loss

Dry mouth and absence of tears

Skin that feels dry and doughy

Eyes that appear sunken

Diminished urine output

Lethargy

HOMEMADE REHYDRATION ELECTROLYTE SOLUTION

1 quart clean water

1/2 teaspoon table salt

1/2 teaspoon baking soda

8 teaspoons sugar

drating electrolyte solution) if your child seems dehyrated. Children often refuse Pedialyte because of the taste. If you make your own rehydrating solution, you can flavor it with a little fruit juice. These solutions should only be used if there are signs of dehydration.

A probiotic supplement can be purchased at any health food store. For breastfeeding babies, 1/4 teaspoon of a powdered *bifidus* formula is appropriate, mixed with breast milk; for older babies, it can be mixed into yogurt or applesauce. Older children should take a 1/4 teaspoon of a powdered lactobacillus formula. Refrigerate all probiotic supplements.

The first homeopathic medicine to use is *Arsenicum album*. If diarrhea

---

Danger Signs with Diarrhea

See a medical provider if any of the following symptoms are present:

Watery or bad smelling stools in a newborn

Severe abdominal pain or bloody stools

Persistent diarrhea that lasts more than forty-eight hours

Vomiting with diarrhea that lasts more than twenty-four hours

---

is persistent, copious, and smelly, switch to *Podophyllum*. These are usually the only home remedies needed.

Acupressure Massage

Try the following acupressure points, to help relieve diarrhea:

Rub the child's thumb from the tip to the base along a line at the lateral edge of the palm surface.

Rub a line on the lateral edge of the forearm (thumb side) from the wrist to the elbow.

Rub a line on the lateral edge of the index finger from the tip to the base.

Massage the point one inch below the knee on the outer side of the shinbone (the acupuncture point Stomach 36).

Earache

Ear infections are grossly overtreated in conventional medical practice. There is very little place for antibiotics in the treatment of ear problems;

certainly they should not be the first treatment of choice. Natural methods are almost always adequate to treat earaches. At least 30 percent of ear infections are viral and will not respond to antibiotics. Bacteria are often resistant to antibiotics. Even doing nothing, an ear infection will usually go away on its own.

Symptoms

Sometimes an earache is preceded by cold symptoms, while other times pain begins suddenly. The discomfort of ear infections can occur anywhere on a scale of minimal to excruciating. Children commonly experience two different types of ear infections. One occurs in the outer ear canal, often after swimming. Water sits in the canal and creates irritation and facilitates the growth of fungus or bacteria. These external canal infections can be prevented in susceptible children by putting a few drops of rubbing alcohol into the ear canal in the evening after swimming to dry out the canal. The other type of infection occurs in the middle ear, behind the eardrum. The eardrum appears red on inspection with an otoscope, and the pain may be severe. Usually these ear infections involve mild discomfort, or pain may be absent entirely. Hearing loss and a feeling of plugged ears are common during ear infections because fluid that collects in the middle ear space blocks the movement of the eardrum. This fluid and the resulting muffled hearing often persist for several weeks, and then resolve on their own.

Parents can easily monitor the color of their child's eardrums with a home otoscope. To purchase one of these inexpensive devices, search for the word otoscope on any Internet search engine. With the otoscope, you are looking for redness of the eardrum. Simply tug the ear backward and outward to straighten out the ear canal, and then gently insert the otoscope tip and look for the grayish-white eardrum. If it looks red, there is probably a middle ear infection. Practice when your child is

---

Danger Signs with Earache

See a medical provider if either of the following symptoms is present:

Discharge or blood from the ear canal (normal earwax is dark orange color)

Persistent fever with ear pain

---

healthy. You can also monitor the recovery of the eardrum by observing the red color fading over a week's time.

Treatment

Place a few drops of room-temperature oil into your child's ear to relieve pain. Olive oil works well. The oil is soothing to the eardrum.

Choose one of the following three homeopathic medicines that best fits the symptoms:

Hepar sulphur for pain that is worse from touch. The child generally likes heat on the ear, but does not want anything touching it and doesn't like having her ears examined. She is irritable and fussy.

Pulsatilla for discomfort that is less intense. The child likes to press on the ear. She is clingy and weepy.

Chamomilla for pain that is severe. The child is very touchy, irritable, and demanding. Pain is worse from warmth.

Vitamin C and Echinacea are appropriate. Use them as you would for colds (see page 222).

Acupressure Massage

Massage the points described to relieve earaches:

Rub the line on the medial edge of the forearm (the pinkie side) from the elbow to the wrist in one direction only.

Rub the palm side of the index finger from the tip toward the base in one direction only.

Massage the two points at the back of the neck in the hollows on either side of the bony prominence at the base of the skull.

Fevers

Fevers, or elevated temperatures, are good. Fever is the body's mechanism for fighting infections—speeding up metabolism to increase heart rate and blood supply where it is needed, producing more white blood cells to devour pathogens, and increasing antibody responses to infection. Fevers should not be suppressed with fever-reducing medication (antipyretics). Acetaminophen, ibuprofen, and aspirin have no place in the home treatment of fevers below 105°F (40.5°C). A child with a fever higher than 105°F should be under medical supervision because a serious infection such as meningitis may be the cause, but only fevers beyond 108°F (42.2°C) have been known to cause brain damage. If your baby under three months of age has a fever or seems sick and lethargic, see your medical provider.

Studies have shown that depriving the body of its ability to develop a fever with antipyretics may prolong the illness, decrease antibody response, and increase the likelihood of disease complications such as pneumonia and meningitis. Medical authorities generally agree that reducing fevers interferes with immune mechanisms and worsens illness. Treating animals with antipyretics during fevers increases their fatality rates.

Many illnesses begin with fevers. Most viral and bacterial infections can stimulate fevers. Sometimes the cause is obvious; at other times, the cause is hidden. For example, urinary tract infections in babies may be characterized by fever without other symptoms. Of course, babies and toddlers cannot tell you their symptoms and it may require a physical exam or even lab tests to determine the cause of an illness. Roseola, a very common childhood viral illness, typically causes a high fever for a few days without other symptoms, and then a rash follows as children recover. For some illnesses in children, fever is the only symptom. Children with a strong immune system may develop a fever to combat an infection and never develop any other typical symptoms of the illness. Some children develop fevers more readily than others, and their temperature may go up with just mild stresses such as exhaustion from an exciting day or mosquito bites.

Seizures can occur with fevers. Some children are more prone to these febrile seizures, and their parents dread the onset of illness. About 50 percent of children who experience one febrile seizure will have another one in the future. Typically, a child will either begin twitching prior to the onset of a seizure, or the seizure will begin suddenly and unexpectedly. If your child begins quivering or trembling, take her into the shower with you immediately. Cooling her down may avert the onset of convulsions. Febrile seizures are frightening to parents even though they only last ten to fifteen seconds, but they do not result in any type of damage to the child. They do not proceed to later epilepsy. If a seizure occurs, keep your child upright if possible and make sure she is breathing well. Reassure her. If she vomits, turn her on her side. Call your medical provider immediately, once the seizure is over. Unless your child is choking or having difficulty breathing, it is usually not necessary to summon emergency services. If your child experiences a febrile seizure, consult with a practitioner of natural medicine to develop a program to prevent future seizures.

DANGER SIGNS WITH FEVER

See a medical provider under the following circumstances:

Any fever in a child under three months of age

Fever reaches 105°F (40.5°C)

Appearance: lethargic, pale skin, unresponsive, weak crying

Symptoms: repeated vomiting, severe headache, stiff neck

Measuring Temperature

The only reasons to measure temperature are to determine if a child is sick, still sick, or developing a dangerously high fever. I do not recommend taking temperatures on a regular basis during illness simply because treatment does not usually depend on what the thermometer says. Other warning signs are much more important in assessing the need for interventions, especially the child's appearance, level of energy, appetite, and severity of symptoms.

There are four commonly used methods, or locations, for measuring body temperature: oral, rectal, ear, and armpit. Ear and rectal temperature readings are equivalent. Oral is lower than the ear or rectal readings, and armpit is lowest. Three types of devices are used for measuring temperature: ear thermometer, digital thermometer, or glass thermometer (with a rectal or oral end). I recommend ear or digital thermometers for home use because there is no danger of breakage and glass fragments. I do not recommend temperature strips (forehead tapes) for measuring temperature.

Although skin temperature is not an especially reliable method of measuring temperature, and children can have fevers without heat in the

TEMPERATURE EQUIVALENTS		
AXILLARY (°F)	ORAL (°F)	RECTAL/EAR (°F)
98.4–99.4	99.4–99.9	100.4–100.9
100–101	101–101.5	102–102.5
101–102	102–102.5	103–103.5
102–103	103–103.5	104–104.5
103–104	104–104.5	105–105.5
AXILLARY (°C)	ORAL (°C)	RECTAL/EAR (°C)
36.9–37.4	37.4–37.7	38–38.3
37.8–38.3	38.3–38.6	38.9–39.2
38.3–38.9	38.9–39.2	39.4–39.7
38.9–39.7	39.4–39.7	40–40.3
39.4–40	40–40.3	40.6–40.8

skin, studies have shown that parents are right 75 percent of the time when estimating whether their child has a fever by feeling the forehead.

The average normal oral temperature is 98.6°F(37°C), but normal temperature readings can vary during the day between 97°F and 100°F. An oral temperature is 0.5°F (0.28°C) to 1°F (0.56°C) lower than a rectal or ear (tympanic) temperature. An armpit (axillary) temperature is usually 0.5°F (0.28°C) to 1°F (0.56°C) lower than an oral temperature.

Treatment
The goals of treating fevers are to encourage the most effective healing

CONVERTING FAHRENHEIT TO CENTIGRADE		
98.6°F	=	37°C
99°F	=	37.2°C
99.5°F	=	37.5°C
99°F	=	37.2°C
100°F	=	37.8°C
100.4°F	=	38°C
101°F	=	38.3°C
102°F	=	38.9°C
103°F	=	39.5°C
104°F	=	40°C
105°F	=	40.6°C
106°F	=	41.1°C
107°F	=	41.7°C

reaction in the body and to make the child comfortable. Start treating fevers in your child with the homeopathic medicine *Belladonna*. If your child is especially droopy, aching, lethargic, and chilly, give *Gelsemium*.

Wiping children with a cool, wet washcloth will cause the water to evaporate from the skin and have a cooling effect. It may not bring down the temperature, but it does provide some relief of symptoms.

If other symptoms accompany the fever, consult those sections in this chapter for additional treatment suggestions. The main problem with fevers is the accompanying headaches that children suffer. See the headache section for suggestions.

Fevers from a viral illness will benefit from several of the same treatment strategies as colds. Vitamin C, Echinacea, and the Chinese herbal formulas Windbreaker or Yin Chao Junior are all appropriate.

Keep your child home from school and resting for twenty-four hours after a fever has subsided. Often children will have a fever in the evening, burn it off in the night, and feel much better in the morning. Then the fever may return later in the afternoon and the child feels droopy again. Better to rest until recovery is complete than to rush back to normal activities and prolong the illness.

Acupressure Massage

Massage the following points to help break a fever:

Massage the ring finger on the palm side from the base to the tip in one direction only.

Massage along a line in the center of the inside of the forearm from the wrist to the elbow in one direction only.

Rub the line on the medial edge of the forearm (the pinkie side) from the elbow to the wrist in one direction only.

Rub the temples in the depression at the outer end of the eyebrows.

Massage the two points at the back of the neck in the hollows on either side of the bony prominence at the base of the skull.

First Aid and Injuries

Strains and Sprains

A **strain** is an injury to tendons or muscles. This is the most common type of overuse injury that arises from twisting or wrenching a mus-

---

DANGER SIGNS WITH SOFT-TISSUE INJURIES

See a medical provider if your child experiences:

Severe pain or swelling at a joint

Inability to use the affected limb

Notable tenderness over an isolated spot in a bone

---

cle. The ankle is the most common site of strains, but other joints can be strained as wellæshoulders, elbows, wrists, or knees. The symptoms are pain and swelling. Bad strains may cause discolorationæredness or bruising.

A **sprain** involves the ligaments that attach bone to bone. The ligament may be stretched or torn, and torn ligaments can be excruciatingly painful, possibly requiring surgery. It may be difficult to tell if a bone is broken. With severe pain or if there is a point of tenderness over a specific spot, there may be a fracture and an x-ray may be required.

Treatment of Strains and Sprains

Home treatment is the same for strains and sprains, and relies on two approaches: first, RICE (as soon as possible after the injury), and second, an appropriate homeopathic remedy.

Step one is RICE (rest, ice, compression, elevation):

Rest—Stay off the injured part. Further motion will aggravate the injury.

Ice—Apply ice (in a plastic bag and wrapped with a towel) or a cold compress to the injured part. This will reduce swelling and bruising; do this three times a day.

Compression—Apply an ace bandage to restrict movement and to reduce swelling; do not use a bandage that cannot stretch.

Elevation—Keep the injured part higher than the heart to prevent swelling.

Step two is an appropriate homeopathic remedy:

As soon as possible following an injury that involves muscles, joints, or bruising, give your child *Arnica*—two pellets every hour for three doses, then every three hours while awake for at least three days. Apply *Arnica* gel to the area two to three times per day. Do not apply *Arnica* externally to skin that is raw from scrapes or cuts.

For sore muscles from sports, use *Arnica* 30 internally and *Arnica* gel externally.

If swelling or pain persists after three days, switch to *Ruta graveolans,* three times per day.

Cuts and Puncture Wounds

Stop the bleeding from a cut by pressing on the wound with a clean cloth, then wash with soap and water. After bleeding has stopped, assess whether stitches may be required. Any cut on the face should be examined professionally. If a cut has gaping edges or is longer than 1/2 inch, consult a medical provider. If there is dirt embedded in a scrape or cut, go to a medical provider to have the wound cleansed.

Step one: *Calendula* tincture in alcohol is usually the only application needed. Dilute the liquid *Calendula* extract (tincture) in a little water, one dropper in 1/4 cup water. Then apply the diluted *Calendula* to the skin. *Calendula* is a natural antiseptic. It stops bleeding, promotes healing of the skin, and prevents infection.

DANGER SIGNS WITH CUTS

See a medical provider if any of the following are present:

Cut longer than 1/2 inch

Redness developing around the cut

Red lines extending up the limb from a cut

Step two: When the wound has healed, apply vitamin E to prevent scarring. Puncture a capsule of vitamin E and apply it to the skin once a day.

Puncture Wounds

The danger associated with puncture wounds is the development of tetanus, a potentially fatal infection caused by bacteria that can only grow in a medium deprived of free oxygen. The tissues and blood vessels beneath the skin can provide just such an environment. Puncture wounds should be allowed to bleed in order to flush out any bacteria injected under the skin. A tetanus-prone wound is a puncture sustained outdoors or an extensive wound with dead tissue.

A tetanus shot may be necessary to prevent this infection. If the initial series of tetanus shots or a booster has been given in the preceding ten years, then a booster shot is not needed. If no tetanus shots have ever been given in the past, then one shot of tetanus immune globulin (TIG) in the emergency room will prevent tetanus from that injury.

Fractures

For any serious injury or persisting pain from an injury, an x-ray may be needed to diagnose a broken bone. If a bone is fractured, an orthopedist will determine the appropriate treatmentæcasting, splinting, or surgery.

Once the fracture has been diagnosed and treated, give *Symphytum* 12C twice a day for six weeks. *Symphytum* (comfrey or boneset) will help the fracture to heal more quickly.

Sunburn and First-Degree Burns

For all burns, immediately run cool tap water over the skin for five to ten minutes. For the redness and discomfort of a sunburn or a mild burn that produces redness, put a few droppers of *Calendula* tincture into 1/2 cup water and apply this to the skin with a cotton ball for small burns or spray it on a sunburn. Aloe vera gel is also a soothing application. Give homeopathic *Urtica urens* every half-hour for several doses.

For more serious burns with blisters, moisture, and seeping, or any white or charred skin, see your medical provider.

Headaches

One of the most common symptoms of school-age children is head pain, second only to stomach aches. Usually headaches are a product of stress, low blood sugar, or a viral illness. Other causes, such as prolonged sun exposure and foods that contain MSG or aspartame, stimulate headaches as well. Migraine headaches are chronic in nature and beyond the scope of acute home prescribing.

Meningitis typically causes severe headaches with vomiting, high fever, stiff neck, disorientation, and lethargy. If you suspect meningitis, contact your medical provider immediately.

Treatment

Give *Belladonna* as the first homeopathic medicine for headaches. If the head pain is made worse by motion or moving the head or eyes and the child has aching muscles and thirst, give *Bryonia*.

Acupressure Massage

An adult or the child himself can apply pressure to the following points to relieve a headache:

The premier point for headaches is Large Intestine 4, the tender spot in the web between the thumb and index finger, squeezed with the thumb and index finger positioned on the front and back of the hand.

Massage the two points at the back of the neck in the hollows on either side of the bony prominence at the base of the skull and two points directly above those.

Rub the temples in the depression at the outer end of the eyebrows.

Rashes and Hives

A rash is characterized by flat pink areas in the skin. It may spread over a wide area, as with diaper rash or viral rashes. Or it may occur in isolated spots, as with hives. Common causes of rashes are allergic reactions, poison oak, viral illness, or heat. Any virus in children, even cold virus, is capable of causing a rash. Some rashes are itchy, some are not. Eczema will cause a rash with dry patches of skin, and sometimes causes cracking, bleeding, and weeping in the skin.

Hives are red blotchy areas, sometimes itchy, that may result from an allergic response or a reaction to a stressful situation. Sometimes the cause of hives in children is never determined. Some foods contain histamine or can stimulate the release of histamine, and result in hives for children who eat them.

If your child experiences a generalized rash with no signs of illness,

---

HISTAMINES AND FOOD

FOODS CONTAINING HISTAMINES:	FOODS RELEASING HISTAMINES:
Fermented cheeses	Egg white
Fish	Chocolate
Shellfish	Strawberries
Spinach	Pork
Tomatoes	

---

the first thing to consider is possible exposure to allergens or skin irritants, either from contact with the skin or ingestion. Some of the most common contact reactions come from laundry detergents, wool, pesticides applied to grass, and poison oak. The most common food allergies in descending order of frequency are eggs, peanuts, milk, fish, soy, and wheat.

Treatment

Give the homeopathic medicine *Urtica urens*, especially if the symptoms are made worse by heat. Give *Rhus tox* if the symptoms are alleviated with heat.

Itching can be relieved by taking a bath with oatmeal powder in the tub. Aveeno packets work well and are available at most drugstores.

Red Eyes

Conjunctivitis, or pinkeye, is an inflammation of the white of the eye, actually the transparent membrane that covers the eyeball. Most instances of conjunctivitis are caused by viruses; rarely is a bacterium involved. Sometimes allergy or exposure to smoke or pollution will cause red eyes.

DANGER SIGNS WITH RED EYES

SEE A MEDICAL PROVIDER IF:

Symptoms persist longer than four or five days

The infection is worsening, or the eye looks cloudy

There is increasing sensitivity to light

Symptoms include itching, burning, or a sensation of sand or dust in the eye. A yellowish discharge may be evident and, in the morning on waking, the eyelids may be stuck together with dried discharge.

Treatment

The only two homeopathic medicines you will need are *Euphrasia* for red, irritated eyes, and *Mercurius (vivus* or *solubilis)* for redness with yellowish discharge from the eyes. Give one or the other.

The best external application for irritated eyes is breast milk. If you are breastfeeding your baby, squirt some into her eyes.

If you have access to a tincture of *Euphrasia,* apply that with a cotton ball. Dilute the *Euphrasia* three droppers in a quarter cup of water. Dip the cotton ball into the solution and wipe the eye from the inner corner to the outer corner, just once. Throw away that cotton ball and use another for several repeated applications. If you do not have *Euphrasia,* use warm water.

Sore Throats

Throat pain accompanies colds, allergies, and strep infections. The tonsils may be swollen, red, and pitted with yellow pus. Lymph nodes below the jaw tend to get swollen as well. Fever and other cold symptoms may also accompany the sore throat. A high fever, as much as 104°F, may signify strep throat, which is generally more severe than viral sore throats, takes longer to go away, and is occasionally accompanied by a rash. In other respects the symptoms can be similar and even indistinguishable unless a throat culture is obtained.

Antibiotics for Strep?

Most pediatricians will insist on treating strep throat with antibiotics. The specific organism is Group A beta-hemolytic streptococcus. The effectiveness of antibiotics for recovery from strep throat has been controversial, with early studies showing no effect on symptoms (Brink et al., 1951; Denny et al., 1953) and later studies showing dramatic improvement (Randolph et al., 1985). The second reason doctors treat strep with antibiotics is because they can prevent one of the complications of strep throat, acute rheumatic fever (ARF), which commonly damages heart valves and can prove fatal. Antibiotics do not seem to prevent some other complications, specifically toxic shock syndrome or kidney infections (Weinstein and Le Frock, 1971). However, the incidence of rheumatic fever has decreased dramatically since the time when thousands of people died every year from that extremely infectious and painful disease. In the late 1940s, 200,000 people per year developed rheumatic fever in the United States. The numbers began declining prior to the availability of antibiotics and ARF has nearly disappeared since the 1970s. Pockets of ARF occur sporadically in various small areas of the country, but rheumatic fever is now largely a disease of the past. Apparently, the strains of the bacteria that have an affinity for attacking the heart simply do not occur anymore except in rare, isolated instances (Markowitz, 1998; Stollerman, 1990). Once upon a time antibiotics prevented ARF that followed strep throat, but now the disease has virtually disappeared, despite the fact that most sore throats do not get treated. In fact, most cases of ARF now have no history of a preceding sore throat.

None of this would be an issue if antibiotics had no side effects. The problem is that they do. Antibiotics disrupt the immune system, and kill beneficial bacteria along with the pathogens. Antibiotics also tend to create resistant strains of bacteria so that they do not work effectively when they are really needed. A further complicating issue is that strep bacteria typically do not disappear from the throat following a course of antibiotics. The bacteria will persist even after signs of the infection have disappeared. If a throat culture is taken at some later date, the bacteria will still be present and another antibiotic prescription will follow even though there is no active infection. Finally, studies have shown that when antibiotics are given for strep throat, the infection tends to recur more often than when they are not prescribed.

I do not recommend antibiotics for strep throat unless an unusual number of ARF cases caused by strep bacteria have been documented in the community, or if your child has pre-existing heart disease. I agree with pediatrician Robert Mendelsohn, whose advice two decades ago remains true today:

> Both throat cultures and antibiotics are to be avoided, because the hazards of treatment outweigh the remote possibility that your child will suffer any lasting effects even if he has a strep infection. (Mendelsohn, 1984)

Treatment

Homeopathic treatment is usually extremely effective in relieving the symptoms of sore throats and stimulating a complete and quick recovery. Strep throat may take longer to resolve than viral sore throats.

Belladonna is the first medicine to prescribe when the throat is inflamed, red, and painful with few other symptoms besides fever.

Mercurius (*vivus* or *solubilis*) is by far the most frequently indicated medicine for children's sore throats. Characteristic symptoms include a bad odor from the mouth, an increase in saliva production with drooling in younger children, swollen lymph nodes, and irritability.

The third medicine is *Phytolacca* when the throat feels swollen or constricted on swallowing and the lymph nodes are swollen, but the typical *Mercurius* symptoms of salivation and bad odor are absent.

Symptomatic treatment includes eating frozen things (juice popsicles or ice chips), sucking on zinc lozenges, and, for older children, gargling with salt water.

Give vitamin C and Echinacea as you would for a cold (see page 222). Give Windbreaker or Yin Chao Junior.

Acupressure Massage

Sore throat pain is alleviated by massaging the following points:

Massage the ring finger on the palm side from the tip to the base in one direction only.

Massage along a line in the center of the inside of the forearm from the wrist to the elbow in one direction only.

Press on a point at the soft junction of the thumb and index finger.

Massage the two points at the back of the neck in the hollows on either side of the bony prominence at the base of the skull.

Styes

If your child has a red bump on the eyelid, it is a benign infection of the oil-secreting glands near the hair follicles. These styes are common in young children and usually go away within a few days. Some children are prone to recurrences and persistent styes. For chronic or recurrent styes, consult your homeopath or natural medicine provider.

Treatment consists of applying warm compresses as often as you can and giving *Pulsatilla*. Usually the stye will fade away. Sometimes styes will form a hard lump in the eyelid and require a different medicine, *Staphysagria*, which may need to be continued for a week or more in order to resolve the problem. *Staphysagria* in a 12C potency once or twice a day should be all that is required.

Teething

Some babies experience more pain with the emergence of teeth than others. In some children, the process of teething is stressful enough to make them cranky and ornery, or sick with colds and fevers. An increase in drooling often occurs with teething, but drooling is common for 6-month-old to 1-year-old children.

If your baby has a bump in the gum that is red and swollen, you know that a tooth is about to emerge. However, it may be hard to tell whether a fussy baby is getting teeth. And teething can be painful without any outward signs in the mouth, just from a tooth pressing through the deeper gums. Stick a finger in your baby's mouth and press on the gum. You may get a reaction if the gum is sensitive.

Treatment

It is helpful to keep some frozen banana in a plastic bag for symptoms of teething. Peel a banana, cut it lengthwise and then in pieces that your baby can hold, and freeze them. The combination of the cold, the soft texture, and the sweetness will produce the desired effect in a form pleasing to babies. Juice popsicles will serve a similar purpose, though you may need to leave them out of the freezer for a few minutes to soften them. You can make these yourself or buy pure frozen juice bars without added sweeteners. (For further suggestions, see page 157.)

Usually the only medicine needed for teething is *Chamomilla*, which can often relieve symptoms immediately. Parents would be wise to keep some on hand for any but the most agreeable and easily comforted babies. I do not recommend combination teething tablets because of the potential for homeopathic medicines that are not appropriate to disrupt a child's delicate energetic balance.

Two Chinese herbal formulas can be very helpful in teething. One is a pediatric formula, Quiet Calm. The other is a general formula, Comfort Shen. Both of these formulas, by Chinese Modular Solutions, have a calming and balancing effect when a child's disturbed equilibrium manifests in emotional outbursts, irritability, and sleeplessness.

Thrush

With thrush, you will see white, cheesy patches inside your baby's mouth on the lips, membranes inside the cheeks, roof of the mouth, or the tongue. These patches differ from the normal white coated tongue of breastfed babies because you cannot just wipe off the patches. Thrush is usually a problem only during the first six months of life. It is caused by Candida albicans, a fungus that is a normal inhabitant of the body. Overgrowth of Candida will produce eruptions in the baby's mouth, in the diaper area, or on a nursing mother's nipples.

Treatment

The first medicine to use is homeopathic *Borax*. You should also give your baby a *bifidus* powder supplement mixed with breast milk or water.

Bifidus bacteria will restore normal intestinal flora in breastfed babies. Several brands of baby *bifidus* formulas in powder form are available at health food stores. Keep the powder refrigerated. Give 1/4 teaspoon per day. Making a solution of the powder and squirting it into your baby's mouth will also help to create an acid environment that discourages growth of the fungus. Do not be discouraged with slow progress. It takes a while for thrush to go away.

A back-up homeopathic medicine for persistent thrush is *Mercurius,* especially if the gums are also red and swollen.

Mothers with thrush on their nipples should take a supplement of mixed intestinal bacteria in capsule form. Add 2–3 drops each of tea tree oil and grapefruit seed extract (available at health food stores) to a lotion or cream and apply it to your nipples. Wash it off prior to nursing. Take non-aged, odor-free garlic tablets that contain at least 3,000 mcg of allicin. For cracked nipples use Lancinoh cream (made from pesticide-free lanolin without preservatives). Stop all sugar-sweetened products in your diet since sugar feeds the fungus.

Vomiting (Stomach Flu and Food Poisoning)

The onset of a viral illness may unexpectedly wake children in the middle of the night with a stomach ache and vomiting. They may vomit repeatedly and become thirsty and then vomit every time they drink. Usually these illnesses are indistinguishable from food poisoning, but both conditions tend to disappear in a day or two. If vomiting persists for more than eight hours or if repeated vomiting will not stop despite your best efforts, call your medical provider.

Some types of vomiting can indicate more serious problems. Projectile vomiting, where the expulsion is forceful and vomit is expelled for some

---

DANGER SIGNS WITH VOMITING

SEE A MEDICAL PROVIDER IF ANY OF THE FOLLOWING OCCUR:

Projectile vomiting

Persistence beyond eight hours

Vomiting with a high fever

Vomiting with increasing abdominal pain

Signs of dehydration—dry eyes and mouth, sunken eyes

---

distance, could indicate an obstruction in the digestive tract. Repeated vomiting with a high fever is a symptom of meningitis. If either of these conditions occurs, call your medical provider immediately.

Treatment

First try to make your child comfortable. A cold wet washcloth on the forehead sometimes stops the vomiting. If your child is having difficulty keeping down fluids, then give only sips of water or ice chips.

The first medicine to use for the onset of vomiting, especially if your child wakes in the night, is *Arsenicum*; repeat every hour or two if necessary. If vomiting persists, switch to homeopathic *Ipecacuanha*. Usually these will be the only medicines required. If other symptoms occur, such as abdominal pain or diarrhea, follow the treatment guidelines in those sections of this chapter.

Acupressure Massage

Massage the following points:

Rub the child's thumb from the tip to the base along a line at the lateral edge of the palm side surface.

Rub a line on the lateral edge (thumb side) of the forearm from the wrist to the elbow.

Massage the point one inch below the knee on the outer side of the shinbone (at the acupuncture point Stomach 36).

REFERENCES

Accardo, J P, et al. Disorders of attention and activity levels in a referral population. *Pediatrics* 1990; 85 (Suppl., Part 2):426–431.

Agency for Toxic Substances and Disease Registry. DEHP, Di(2-ethylhexyl) phthalate. *ToxFAQs* April 1993.

Ala-Houhala, M, et al. Maternal compared with infant vitamin D supplementation. *Archives of Diseases in Childhood* 1986; 61:1159–1163.

American Academy of Allergy, Asthma and Immunology. Bronchospasm in competitive swimmers. Presented at the 57th Annual Meeting 03/20/2001.

American Academy of Pediatrics Work Group on Cow's Milk Protein and Diabetes Mellitus. Infant feeding practices and their possible relationship to the etiology of diabetes mellitus. *Pediatrics* 1994 Nov; 94(5):752–754.

American Conference of Governmental Industrial Hygienists (ACGIH). *Documentation of the threshold limit values and biological exposure indices.* 6th ed. Cincinnati, Ohio: ACGIH, 1991.

Anderson, C, and Dill, K. Video games and aggressive thoughts, feelings, and behavior in the laboratory and in life. *Journal of Personality and Social Psychology* 2000; 78(4):772–790.

Anderson, I. Showers pose a risk to health. *New Scientist* 1986, August 18.

Armstrong, Thomas. *The Myth of the A.D.D. Child: 50 Ways to Improve Your Child's Behavior and Attention Span without Drugs, Labels, or Coercion.* New York: Plume, 1997.

Bee, G. Dietary conjugated linoleic acids alter adipose tissue and milk lipids of pregnant and lactating sows. *Journal of Nutrition* 2000; 130:2292–2298.

Blumenthal, et al. *The Complete German Commission E Monographs, Therapeutic Guide to Herbal Medicines.* The American Botanical Council, Austin, Texas, and Integrative Medicine Communications, Boston, Mass., 1998.

Brink, W R, et al. Effect of penicillin and aureomycin on natural course of streptococcal tonsillitis and pharyngitis. *American Journal Medicine* 1951; 297:365.

Butte, N F, et al. *Nutrient adequacy of exclusive breastfeeding for the term infant during the first six months of life.* Geneva: World Health Organization, 2002, pp. 26–30.

Calvani, M, et al. Fever episodes in early life and the development of atopy in children with asthma. *European Respiratory Journal* 2002 Aug; 20(2):391–396.

Carroll-Pankhurst, C, and Mortimer, A. Sudden infant death syndrome, bed-sharing, parental weight, and age at death. *Pediatrics* 2001; 107(3):530–536.

Chong, D S, et al. Maternal smoking: an increasing unique risk factor for sudden infant death syndrome in Sweden. *Acta Paediatr.* 2004 Apr; 93(4):471–478.

Christakis, D A. Early television exposure and subsequent attentional problems in children. *Pediatrics* 2004 Apr; 113(4):708–713.

Cohet, C, et al. Infections, medication use, and the prevalence of symptoms of asthma, rhinitis, and eczema in childhood. *J Epidemiology Community Health* 2004 Oct; 58(10):852–857.

Cohn, P D. *An Epidemiological Report on Drinking Water: Fluoridation and Osteosarcoma in Young Males,* Trenton: New Jersey Department of Health, Environmental Health Service, November 8, 1992.

Collins, R L, et al. Watching sex on television predicts adolescent initiation of sexual behavior. *Pediatrics* 2004 Sep; 114(3):e280–289.

Colon, I, et al. Identification of phthalate esters in the serum of young Puerto Rican girls with premature breast development. *Environmental Health Perspectives* 2000 Jul; 112(10):A541–543.

Connor, W E, et al. Increased docosahexaenoic acid levels in human newborn infants by administration of sardines and fish oil during pregnancy. *Lipids* 1996; 31(suppl):S183–187.

Curl, C L, Fenske, R A, and Elgethun, K. Organophosphorus pesticide exposure of urban and suburban preschool children with organic and conventional diets. *Environmental Health Perspectives* 2003; 111(3).

Davies, D P. Cot death in Hong Kong: a rare problem? *Lancet* 1985; 2:1346–1348.

Denny, F W, et al. Comparative effects of penicillin, aureomycin and terramycin on streptococcal tonsillitis and pharyngitis. *Pediatrics* 1953; 11:7.

Diesendorf, D. The mystery of declining tooth decay. *Nature* 1986; 322:125–129.

Divi, R L, et al. Anti-thyroid isoflavones from soybean: isolation, characterization, and mechanisms of action. *Biochemical Pharmacology* 1997 Nov; 54(10):1087–1096.

Douglas, et al. Impact of water fluoridation on dental practices and dental manpower. *Journal of the American Dental Assoc.* 1972; 84:355–367.

Droste, J H, et al. Does the use of antibiotics in early childhood increase the risk of asthma and allergic disease? *Clinical Exper Allergy* 2000 Nov; 30(11):1547–1553.

Duty, S M, et al. Phthalate exposure and human semen parameters. *Epidemiology* 2003(a) May; 14(3):269–277.

Duty, S M, et al. The relationship between environmental exposures to phthalates and DNA damage in human sperm using the neutral comet assay. *Environmental Health Perspectives* 2003 Jul; 111(9):1164–1169.

Fallon, S, and Enig, M. *Nourishing Traditions,* Washington, DC: NewTrends Publishing, 2001.

Fidler N, et al. Docosahexaenoic acid transfer into human milk after dietary supplementation: a randomized clinical trial. *Journal of Lipid Research,* 2000 Sept; 41:1376–1383.

Fomon, S J, Ekstrand, J, and Ziegler, E E. Fluoride intake and prevalence of dental fluorosis: trends in fluoride intake with special attention to infants. *Journal of Public Health Dentistry* 2000; 60:131–139.

Forsyth, J S, et al. Relation between early introduction of solid food to infants and their weight and illnesses during the first two years of life. *British Medical Journal* 1993 Jun 12; 306(6892):444.

Fort, P, et al. Breast feeding and insulin-dependent diabetes mellitus in children. *Journal American College Nutrition* 1986; 5(5):439.

Fort, P, et al. Breast and soy-formula feedings in early infancy and the prevalence of autoimmune thyroid disease in children. *Journal American College Nutrition* 1990 Apr; 9(2):164–167.

Francois, C A, et al. Supplementing lactating women with flaxseed oil does not increase docosahexaenoic acid in their milk. *American Journal Clinical Nutrition* 2003 Oct; 78(4):806.

Freni-Titulaer, L W, et al. Premature thelarche in Puerto Rico: a search for environmental factors. *American Journal Diseases of Children* 1986 Dec; 140(12):1263–1267.

Fukai, S, and Hiroshi, F. *1999 Annual Report, Japan SIDS Family Association*, Sixth SIDS International Conference, Auckland, New Zealand, 2000.

Gartner, L M, et al. Prevention of rickets and vitamin D deficiency: new guidelines for vitamin D intake. *Pediatrics* 2003 Apr; 111(4):908–910.

Gemmel, A, et al. Blood lead level and dental caries in school-age children. *Environmental Health Perspectives* 2002; 110(10):A625–630.

Gerard, C M, et al. Spntaneous arousals in supine infants while swaddled and unswaddled during rapid eye movement and quiet sleep. *Pediatrics* 2002 Dec; 100(6):e70.

Gillman, M W, et al. Risk of overweight among adolescents who were breastfed as infants. *Journal American Medical Association.* 2001; 285(19):2461–2467.

Glerup, H, et al. Commonly recommended daily intake of vitamin D is not sufficient if sunlight exposure is limited. *Journal Internal Medicine* 2000, 247(2): 260–268.

Good Mojab, C. Sunlight deficiency and breastfeeding. *Breastfeeding Abstracts* 2002; 22(1):3–4.

Hanson, L A. Breastfeeding provides passive and likely long-lasting active immunity. *Annals Allergy Asthma Immunology* 1998; 81(6):523–533.

Hardell, L, and Eriksson, M. A case-control study of non-Hodgkin lymphoma and exposure to pesticides. *Cancer* 1999; 85(6):1353–1360.

Hileman, B. New studies cast doubt on fluoridation benefits. *Chemical & Engineering News.* 1989; May 8.

Horwood, L J, and Fergusson, D M. Breastfeeding and later cognitive and academic outcomes. *Pediatrics* 1998; 101:1–7.

Hunt, P, et al. Bisphenol A exposure causes meiotic aneuploidy in the female mouse. *Current Biology* 2003 Apr; 13(1): 546–553.

Hurwitz, E L, and Morgenstern, H. Effects of diphtheria-tetanus-pertussis or tetanus vaccination on allergies and allergy-related respiratory symptoms among children and adolescents in the US. *Journal Manipulative and Physiological Therapeutics* 2000; 318(7192):1173–1176.

Hyland, G J. Physics and biology of mobile telephony. *Lancet* 2000 Nov 25; 356(9244):1782–1783.

Institute of Medicine, Food and Nutrition Board. *Dietary Reference Intakes: Calcium, Phosphorus, Magnesium, Vitamin D and Fluoride.* Washington, DC: National Academy Press, 1999.

Irvine, C H G, et al. The potential adverse effects of soybean phyto-estrogens in infant feeding. *New Zealand Medical Journal* 1995; 24:318.

Jensen, C L, et al. Effect of docosahexaenoic acid supplementation of lactating women on the fatty acid composition of breast milk lipids and maternal and infant plasma phospholipids. *American Journal Clinical Nutrition* 2000 Jan; 71(suppl):S292–299.

Karjalainen, J, et al. A bovine albumin peptide as a possible trigger of insulin-dependent diabetes mellitus. *New England Journal Medicine* 1992; 327:302–307.

Kembra, L H, et al. Bisphenol A is released from used polycarbonate animal cages into water at room temperature. *Environmental Health Perspectives* 2003; 111(9).

Kemp, T, Pearce, N, Fitzharris, P, et al. Is infant immunization a risk factor for childhood asthma or allergy? *Epidemiology* 1997; 8:678.

Kibel, M A, and Davies, M F. Should the infant sleep in mother's bed? *Program and Abstracts, Sixth SIDS International Conference, Auckland, New Zealand,* February 8–11, 2000.

Kostraba, J N, et al. Early exposure to cow's milk and solid foods in infancy, genetic predisposition, and risk of IDDM. *Diabetes* 1993; 42:288–295.

Kundi, M, et al. Mobile telephones and cancer—a review of epidemiological evidence. *Journal Toxicology and Environmental Health Part B: Critical Reviews* 2004 Sep-Oct; 7(5):351–384.

Lee, L. *The Enzyme Cure*. Alternativemedicine.com books, 1998.

Lee, N P, et al. Sudden infant death syndrome in Hong Kong: confirmation of low incidence. *British Medical Journal* 1999; 298:72.

Li, X S, et al. Effects of fluoride exposure on the intelligence of children. *Fluoride* 1995; 28:182–189.

Linn, S. *Consuming Kids: The Hostile Takeover of Childhood*. New Press, 2004.

Markowitz, M. Rheumatic fever—a half-century perspective. *Pediatrics* 1998; 102(1)Suppl.:272–274.

Marshall, S J, et al. Relationships between media use, body fatness and physical activity in children and youth: a meta-analysis. *International Journal Obesity* 2004 Oct; 28(10):1238–1246.

Martin, R P, and Holbrook, J. Relationship of temperament characteristics to the academic achievement of first-grade children. *Journal Psychoeducational Assessment* 1985; 3:377–386.

Mendelsohn, R. *How to Raise a Healthy Child... In Spite of Your Doctor*. Contemporary Books, 1984, p. 120.

Mercola, J. The proven danger of microwaves. *NEXUS Magazine*, 1995 Apr-May; 2(25).

Merlino, L A, et al. Vitamin D intake is inversely associated with rheumatoid arthritis: results from the Iowa women's health study. *Arthritis & Rheumatism* 2004; 50(1): 72–77.

Milner, J D, et al. Early infant multivitamin supplementation is associated with increased risk for food allergy and asthma. *Pediatrics* 2004 Jul; 114:27–32.

Mitchell, E A, et al. Clinical characteristics and serum essential fatty acid levels in hyperactive children. *Clinical Pediatrics* 1987; 26:406–411.

Morgan, J, et al. Eczema and early solid feeding in preterm infants. *Archives Diseases of Childhood* 2004 Apr; 89(4):295.

Mortensen, E L, et al. The association between duration of breastfeeding and adult intelligence. *Journal American Medical Association* 2002; 287:2365–2371.

Munger, K L, et al. Vitamin D intake and incidence of multiple sclerosis. *Neurology* 2004; 62(1):60–65.

Murata, K, et al. Delayed brainstem auditory evoked potential latencies in 14 year old children exposed to methylmercury. *Journal Pediatrics,* 2004 Feb; 144(2):177–183.

Mustchin, C P, and Pickering, C A. "Coughing water": bronchial hyper-reactivity induced by swimming in a chlorinated pool. *Thorax* 1979; 34(5):682–683.

National Academy of Sciences. *Neurotoxins: At Home and the Workplace (Report by the Committee on Science and Technology. US House of Representatives, Sept. 16, 1986).* Report 99-827.

Nelson, E A S, et al. International child care practice study: infant sleeping environment. *Early Human Development* 2001; 62:43–55.

Ness, C. Organic label muddies the waters. *San Francisco Chronicle*: April 28, 2004.

Neustaedter, R. *The Vaccine Guide: Risks and Benefits for Children and Adults.* Berkeley, Calif.: North Atlantic Books, 2002.

Norris, J M, et al. Timing of initial cereal exposure in infancy and risk of islet autoimmunity. *Journal American Medical Association* 2003; 290:1713–1720.

Noverr, M C, et al. Role of antibiotics and fungal microbiota in driving pulmonary allergic responses. *Infectious Immunology* 2004 Sep; 72(9):4996–5003.

Odent, M R, Culpin, E E, and Kimmel, T. Letter to the editor. Pertussis vaccination and asthma: is there a link? *Journal American Medical Association* 1994; 272:592–593.

Oddy, W H, et al. Breastfeeding and cognitive development in childhood: a prospective birth cohort study. *Paediatric Perinatology Epidemiology* 2003; 1:81–90.

Oddy, W H, et al. The relation of breastfeeding and body mass index to asthma and atopy in children: a prospective cohort study to age 6 years. *American Journal Public Health* 2004; 94(9):1531–1537.

Paul, I A, et al. Effect of dextromethorphan, diphenhydramine, and placebo on nocturnal cough and sleep quality for coughing children and their parents. *Pediatrics* 2004 Jul; 114:e85–e90.

Pesticide Residues Committee. *Pesticide Residues Monitoring Report: Fourth Quarter Report, 2003.* Available at http://www.pesticides.gov.uk/prc.asp?id=1223.

Randolph, M F, et al. Effect of antibiotic therapy on the clinical course of streptococcal pharyngitis. *Journal Pediatrics* 1985; 106(6):870–875.

Reddy, N R, and Sathe, S K, eds. *Food Phytates,* Boca Raton, Fla.: CRC Press, 2002.

Richard, C. Sleeping position, orientation, and proximity in bedsharing infants and mothers. *Sleep* 1996; 19(9):685–690.

Sanchez-Echaniz, J, et al. Methemoglobinemia and consumption of vegetables in infants. *Pediatrics* 2001 May; 107(5):1024–1028.

Santti, R, et al. Phytoestrogens: potential endocrine disrupters in males. *Toxicol Environmental Health* 1998; 14(1-2):223-237.

Sarveiya, V, et al. Liquid chromatographic assay for common sunscreen agents: application to in vivo assessment of skin penetration and systemic absorption in human volunteers. *Journal Chromatogr B Analyt Technol Biomed Life Sci* 2004 Apr; 803(2):225–231.

Sharpe, R M, et al. Infant feeding with soy formula milk: Effects on the testis and on blood testosterone levels in marmoset monkeys during the period of neonatal testicular activity. *Human Reproduction* 2002; 17(7):1692–1703.

Sprott, T J. *The Cot Death Cover-Up?* Auckland, New Zealand: Penguin Books, 1996.

Stallone, D D, and Jacobson, M F. Cheating babies: nutritional quality and cost of commercial baby food. *Center for Science in the Public Interest (CSPI) Reports,* 1995.

Stevens, L J, et al. Essential fatty acid metabolism in boys with attention-deficit hyperactivity disorder. *American Journal Clinical Nutrition* 1995;62:761–768.

Stevens, L J, et al. Omega-3 fatty acids in boys with behavior, learning, and health problems. *Physiol Behavior* 1996 Apr-May; 59(4–5):915–20.

Stitt, P. *Fighting the Food Giant.,* Natural Press, 1983.

Stollerman, G H. Rheumatogenic group A streptococci and the return of rheumatic fever. *Advances Internal Medicine* 1990; 35:1–25.

Strasburger, V C. Does television affect learning and school performance? *Pediatrician* 1986; 38:141–147.

Strasburger, V C. *Children, Adolescents, and the Media*. SAGE Publications, 2002.

Tappin, D, et al. Used infant mattresses and sudden infant death syndrome in Scotland: case-control study. *British Medical Journal* 2002; 325:1007.

Thoman, E B, and Graham, S E. Self-regulation of stimulation by premature infants. *Pediatrics* 1986; 78:855–860.

U.S. Environmental Protection Agency. Risk Assessment Forum, Washington, DC. *Supplemental Guidance for Assessing Cancer Susceptibility from Early-Life Exposure to Carcinogens*. External Review Draft, EPA/630/R-03/003, 2003.

Vieth, R, et al. Efficacy and safety of vitamin D3 intake exceeding the lowest observed adverse effect level. *American Journal Clinical Nutrition* 2001; 73(2):288–294.

Watkins, B A, and Seifert, M F. Food lipids and bone health, in *Food Lipids and Health*, McDonald, R E, and Min, E B, eds. New York: Marcel Dekker, Inc., 1996.

Watts, M. Roundup and cancer. *Soil & Health* 1998; 58(3):16.

Weinstein, L, and Le Frock, J. Does antimicrobial therapy of streptococcal pharyngitis or pyoderma alter the risk of glomerulonephritis? *Journal Infectious Diseases* 1971; 124(2): 229–231.

Winter, J S D, et al. Pituitary-gonadal relations in infancy: patterns of serum gonadal steroid concentrations in man from birth to two years of age. *Journal Clinical Edocrinological Metabolism* 1976; 42:679–686.

Yelland, J, et al. Explanatory models about maternal and infant health and sudden infant death syndrome among Asian-born mothers, in *Asian Mothers, Australian Birth, Pregnancy, Childbirth, Child Rearing: The Asian Experience in an English-Speaking Country*, Rice, P L, ed. Melbourne: Ausmeed Publications, 1996, pp. 175–189.

Ziegler, A-G, et al. Early infant feeding and risk of developing type 1 diabetes-associated autoantibodies. *Journal American Medical Association* 2003; 290:1721–1728.

Zutavern, A, et al. The introduction of solids in relation to asthma and eczema. *Archives Diseases of Childhood* 2004 Apr; 89(4):303–308.

Home Medicine Kit

Common Homeopathic Medicines

Aconitum

Allium cepa

Antimonium crudum

Arnica

Arsenicum

Belladonna

Bryonia

Chamomilla

Colocynth

Euphrasia

Gelsemium

Hepar sulphur

Ipecacuanha

Kali bichromicum

Ledum

Mercurius

Nux vomica

Phytolacca

Podophyllum

Pulsatilla

Rhus tox

Rumex crispus

Ruta graveolans

Urtica urens

Calendula tincture

Chinese Herbal Formulas

Chinese Modular Solutions (available to practitioners from K'An Herbs, www.kanherbs.com or 800-543-5233):

Chest Relief

Fire Fighter

Windbreaker

Yin Chao Junior (available to practitioners from Health Concerns, 800-233-9355)

A Parent's Library: Recommended Books

Breastfeeding

The Womanly Art of Breastfeeding by La Leche League International (Plume Books, 2004). Still the classic instruction manual that promotes the virtues and presents the nitty-gritty of how to do it. Updated with scientific information.

The Breastfeeding Book by Martha and William Sears (Little, Brown, 2000). Similar information contained in *The Baby Book* by the Sears team; provides everything you need to be successful, with an emphasis on bedsharing, attachment parenting, and extended breastfeeding.

The Ultimate Breastfeeding Book of Answers by Jack Newman and Teresa Pitman (Prima Lifestyles, 2000). Written by another world-renowned pediatrician who specializes in breastfeeding, this guide takes you through all the steps necessary to establish a healthy breastfeeding relationship and answers an amazing number of practical, obscure, and unusual questions about breastfeeding details.

The Nursing Mother's Herbal by Sheila Humphrey (Fairview Press, 2004). Written by a lactation consultant and La Leche League leader, this book covers safety of herbs, therapeutic uses for milk, production problems and breast problems, and suggestions for success in lactation.

Nutrition

Super Baby Food by Ruth Yaron (F. J. Roberts Pub., 1998). Full of valuable advice about the introduction of solid foods through the toddler years. Emphasis is on organic foods and a vegetarian diet. The sections on preparation of foods are excellent, but the emphasis on avoidance of bacteria and her advice about fats require some critical reading.

Nourishing Traditions: The Cookbook that Challenges Politically Correct Nutrition and the Diet Dictocrats by Sally Fallon with Mary Enig (New Trends Publishing, 2001). An excellent theoretical and practical book about nutrition and cooking, with over 700 recipes. As the authors say, "a fascinating guide to wise food choices and proper preparation techniques," recalling the culinary customs of our ancestors. This is the book I wholeheartedly recommend for family nutrition.

The Family Nutrition Book: Everything You Need to Know About Feeding Your Children from Birth Through Adolescence by William and Martha Sears (Little, Brown, 1999). You'll learn how the body works, how to read food labels, what ingredients to look for (and which to avoid), what are thought to prevent cancer, and more. The Searses also offer helpful food lists: good fats, best proteins, and top 10 complex carbohydrates. One caveat: Their thinking on fats is outdated and needs revising.

Eat Healthy, Feel Great by William and Martha Sears (Little, Brown, 2002). Written for elementary school children, this little book presents the tools kids need to make their own wise food choices.

The School Lunchbox Cookbook by Miriam Jacobs (Globe Pequot Press, 2003). Everything you need to know to pack healthy lunches for your kids.

Home Prescribing

Everybody's Guide to Homeopathic Medicines by Dana Ullman and Stephen Cummings (Jeremy P. Tarcher, 1997), and *Homeopathic Medicine for Children & Infants* by Dana Ullman (JP Tarcher, 1992). The classics for quick homeopathic prescribing for acute ailments.

Homeopathic Self-Care: The Quick and Easy Guide for the Whole Family by Robert Ullman and Judyth Reichenberg-Ullman (Prima Publishing,

1997). A homeopathic home prescriber with step-by-step instructions and carefully constructed visual presentations in a graphic format that proceeds logically and simply to guide choices to the correct medicine.

The Homeopathic Emergency Guide by Thomas Kruzel (North Atlantic Books, 1992). This is the best supplementary book for detailed homeopathic descriptions of acute symptoms that will help to differentiate the alternative prescriptions.

Smart Medicine for a Healthier Child: A Practical A–Z Reference to Natural and Conventional Treatments for Infants and Children by Janet Zand and Robert Rountree (Avery Publishing Group, 2003). This book contains extended discussions of each symptom or disease in alphabetic order with corresponding conventional and alternative treatment methods (homeopathy, herbs, and acupressure).

Bedsharing

Good Nights: The Happy Family's Guide to the Family Bed (And a Peaceful Night's Sleep) by Jay Gordon (St. Martin's Press, 2002).

Three in a Bed—The Benefits of Sharing Your Bed with Your Baby by Deborah Jackson (Bloomsbury, 1999).

Nighttime Parenting—How to Get Your Baby and Child to Sleep by William Sears and Mary White. (La Leche League International, 1999).

The Family Bed by Tine Thevenin (Avery Publishing Group, 1987).

Parenting

The Baby Book: Everything You Need to Know About Your Baby from Birth to Age Two by William and Martha Sears (Little, Brown, 2003). One of the best how-to baby books with a baby-centered approach to promoting attachment. All of the Searses' books encourage a natural and healthy lifestyle. I also recommend their *Pregnancy Book, Birth Book, Breastfeeding Book*, and *Family Nutrition Book*. Be warned, however, that the medical advice follows established, conventional pediatrician guidelines.

Natural Family Living by Peggy O'Mara (Pocket Books, 2000). Contains a wealth of information about the distinctive style of parenting promoted by *Mothering Magazine,* Ms. O'Mara's publication. She briefly discusses alternative medicine for children, but the majority of the book is devoted to psychological and developmental issues. She includes no specific information about treating medical problems.

Attachment Parenting: Instinctive Care for your Baby and Young Child by Katie Allison Granju (Atria, 1999). Techniques to facilitate connection and communication are outlined, but mostly the book is an exhortation to listen and to *trust* yourself, and to trust your child's ability to convey to you what he or she needs.

The Difficult Child

Transforming the Difficult Child: The Nurtured Heart Approach by Howard Glasser (Center for the Difficult Child, 1999). Clear and simple techniques for changing the dynamic in your home and the heart of your child.

The Difficult Child by Stanley Turecki (Bantam, 2000).

The Challenging Child: Understanding, Raising, and Enjoying the Five "Difficult" Types of Children by Stanley Greenspan (Perseus Books Group, 1996). The familiar emotional stages of childhood are translated here into types of behavior issues that parents find the most difficult to manage.

Children the Challenge by Rudolf Dreikurs (Plume Books, 1991). This classic establishes a parenting style built on natural consequences and builds a framework for managing the wide range of discipline problems with compassion, consistency, and love.

Rage-Free Kids: Homeopathic Medicine for Defiant, Aggressive, and Violent Children by Judyth Reichenberg-Ullman and Robert Ullman (Prima Lifestyles, 1999). The homeopathic alternative to drug management of behavior problems described by two experts in the field of holistic and homeopathic pediatrics.

Learning

A Mind at a Time (Simon & Schuster, 2003) and *The Myth of Laziness* (Simon & Schuster, 2003) by Mel Levine . These two books set forth Dr. Levine's now famous approach to learning problems that involves identifying children's strengths and weaknesses in learning skills and fostering self-esteem by focusing on their strengths. Parents can identify children's learning styles and help them overcome learning differences. The sequel identifies children's "output problems" that often lead to avoidance behaviors and the label of laziness.

All Kinds of Minds (Educators Publishing Service, 1993) and *Keeping a Head in School* (Educators Publishing Service, 1990) by Mel Levine. These two books help children learn about the way their minds work. The first depicts several students who are having learning problems. It is designed to help children under 11 understand learning differences. The second book, written for children over 11, describes the basic learning skills and attention so they can discover their own strengths and weaknesses in learning.

Beyond ADD: Hunting for Reasons in the Past and Present (Underwood Books, 1996) and *Understanding ADD: A Different Perception* (Underwood Books, 1997) by Thom Hartmann. Both books describe Hartmann's understanding of the value of ADD characteristics as creative, adventurous ways of exploring the world and making discoveries and innovations. A different perception indeed.

In Their Own Way: Discovering and Encouraging Your Child's Multiple Intelligences (Jeremy. P. Tarcher, 2000), *The Myth of the A.D.D. Child: 50 Ways to Improve Your Child's Behavior and Attention Span without Drugs, Labels, or Coercion* (Plume Books, 1997), and *Awakening Your Child's Natural Genius: Enhancing Curiosity, Creativity, and Learning Ability* (Jeremy. P. Tarcher, 1991), by Thomas Armstrong. Armstrong has been writing for decades about the principles of multiple intelligence, the myth of ADD diagnoses, and the ways to stimulate creativity and a fascination with learning. Also see www.thomasarmstrong.com.

Ritalin-Free Kids: Safe and Effective Homeopathic Medicine for ADD and Other Behavioral and Learning Problems by Judyth Reichenberg-Ullman and Robert Ullman (Three Rivers Press, 2000). The homeopathic alternative to the highly toxic drug treatment inflicted on children to manage ADD and behavior problems, written by two experts in the field of holistic and homeopathic pediatrics.

Environment and Chemical Exposure

Chemical-Free Kids: How to Safeguard Your Child's Diet and Environment by Allan Magaziner et al. (Twin Streams Books, 2003). Excellent discussions of pesticides, fake and toxic foods, avoiding toxins in the home environment, and eating organic foods, with many recipes for children's meals and snacks.

Guide to Natural Baby Care: Nontoxic and Environmentally Friendly Ways to Take Care of Your New Child by Mothers and Others for a Livable Planet, Mindy Pennybacker and Aisha Ikramuddin (John Wiley & Sons, 1999). Thousands of suggestions for raising children in natural, nontoxic, and environmentally friendly surroundings. Covers baby equipment, pollutants in the home, babyproofing, and more.

*Our Stolen Future: Are We Theatening our Fertility,Intelligence, and Survival?
A Scientific Detective Story,* by Thea Colborn et al. (Penguin Books, 1997). An in-depth examination of the role of industrial pollutants as hormone disruptors that cause hormone-related cancers, endometriosis, and fertility disorders.

The Fluoride Deception by Christopher Bryson (Seven Stories Press, 2004). The shocking story of how a secretive group of powerful industries abused their influence and power to foist one of the most damaging environmental pollutants of the Cold War era on an unsuspecting and deluded public, managing to get this toxic chemical added to drinking water and toothpaste.

Home Safe Home: Protecting Yourself and Your Family from Everyday Toxics and Harmful Household Products in the Home by Debra Lynn Dadd (Jeremy P. Tarcher, 1997). Simple suggestions to replace toxic products with simple, natural, do-it-yourself formulas.

Vaccination

The Vaccine Guide: Risks and Benefits for Children and Adults by Randall Neustaedter (North Atlantic Books, 2002). All the information that parents need to make a truly informed decision that considers adverse effects and efficacy connected with vaccines, and disease incidence and complications. Adults will find useful chapters on travel vaccines and newer vaccines for possible terrorist attacks.

Websites

This section outlines the goals and visions of websites that provide supportive materials and services for parents who seek to make informed decisions. Information is courtesy of the Holistic Pediatric Association.

Attachment Parenting International:

http://www.attachmentparenting.org

Attachment Parenting International (API) is a nonprofit member organization, networking with parents, professionals, and like-minded organizations around the world. In addition to providing assistance in forming attachment parenting support groups, API functions as a clearinghouse for educational materials, research information, and consultative, referral, and speaker services to promote attachment parenting concepts.

Birthing the Future®:

http://www.birthingthefuture.com

The mission of Birthing the Future, a nonprofit organization, is to gather, synthesize, and disseminate the "finest world wisdom that inspires people about the significance of birthing in each of our lives." The organization focuses upon "what is ideal for mothers and babies that will promote their physical, psychological, and spiritual well-being and the development of their full potential, in the context of family, community, and society."

Breastfeeding.com:

http://www.breastfeeding.com

"You know breastfeeding is a good thing, and you think more people ought to know about it? You have found the right place. Here you will find the best breastfeeding articles on the web. Most articles are of general interest."

Cure-Guide.com:

http://www.cure-guide.com

Dr. Neustaedter's website contains registration for a free email newsletter with updates on pediatric topics, vaccine issues, and influenza, as well as reviews of new health research that affects adults.

Families for Natural Living:

http://www.familiesfornaturalliving.org

Families for Natural Living is a nonprofit educational organization and grassroots network, "by parents for parents who want to make conscious, compassionate, and informed choices for their children. FNL connects and supports parents to create their own natural living community groups." Visitors can find or start a local FNL group on the website or by calling a hotline at 888-FNL-GRPS.

Healthy Child Online:

http://www.healthychild.com

Healthy Child Online is a parenting website that publishes an e-newsletter with reliable information about natural health and holistic medicine for children. The site offers insights on "encouraging and fostering in children the following qualities: self-love, compassion for others, joy, contentment, and vibrant health and vitality on all levels—physical, mental, emotional, and spiritual." Healthy Child Online also provides parents and caregivers free information on safe, natural products to enhance the health and lives of children.

Holistic Moms Network:

http://www.holisticmoms.org

The Holistic Moms Network is a national nonprofit support and resource network for "moms interested in natural and alternative health and mindful parenting." Visitors will find support for building "local holistic communities or chapters that will provide them with a happy, healthy forum for their mothering styles and which will bring them together in an environment that respects their parenting choices."

Holistic Pediatric Association:

http://www.hpakids.org

Nonprofit educational website providing information and support to parents and pediatric health professionals in holistic medicine and natural parenting. Focuses on helping parents reduce the use of ineffective and harmful drug treatments and build healthy bodies and spirits in their children. Visitors can search the HPA Health Professional Directory for a local holistic practitioner and have access to a free holistic parenting e-newsletter, parenting forums, and hundreds of holistic health articles.

Inspired Parenting:

http://www.inspiredparenting.net

A web community providing information and inspiration for everyone who is interested in working with children: grandparents, parents, caregivers, teachers, and others. The network focuses on children who are in late toddlerhood through elementary school, and offers "mindbody approaches for parenting the whole child, which includes support for children's physical health, emotions, mental development, and spirit."

International Chiropractic Pediatric Association:

http://www.icpa4kids.org

The International Chiropractic Pediatric Association is dedicated to advancing awareness of the "chiropractic family wellness lifestyle," through education, training, and research in the care of children and pregnant women.

La Leche League:

http://www.lalecheleague.org

La Leche League was founded to give information and encouragement, mainly through personal help, to mothers who want to breastfeed their babies. While complementing the care of the physician and other health care profession-

als, the organization "recognizes the unique importance of one mother help-ing another to perceive the needs of her child and to learn the best means of fulfilling those needs."

Liedloff Continuum Network:

http://www.continuum-concept.org

The Liedloff Continuum Network (LCN) educates and serves the public—"especially parents, parents-to-be, and anyone who cares about the well-being of infants and children, by advocating the principles described in the book The Continuum Concept and suggesting practical ways to integrate them into daily life." The network also serves people who are "recovering from the adverse effects of a modern, 'non-continuum' upbringing."

Dr. Mercola's Health Newsletter:

http://www.mercola.com

Mercola.com provides guidance on the "best nutrition, medical, emotional therapy, and lifestyle choices to improve and maintain total health. It is Dr. Mercola's vision to transform the existing medical paradigm from one addicted to pharmaceuticals, surgeries and other methods that only conceal or remove specific symptoms—with morbid results to our health and economy—to one focused on treating and preventing the underlying causes." This site has excellent search capabilities for information on the problems with soy, milk, wheat, and other challenges that face parents who want the best nutrition for their children.

Mothering Magazine:

http://www.mothering.com

Mothering Magazine "celebrates the experience of parenthood as worthy of one's best efforts and fosters awareness of the immense importance and value of parenthood and family life in the development of the full human potential."

Each issue contains philosophical inspiration and practical advice about family living. Topics are as diverse as circumcision, vaccinations, organic foods, childhood illnesses, home birth, ear infections, parenting teens, website information, midwifery, and homeopathy.

National Organization of Circumcision Information Resource Centers (NOCIRC):

http://www.nocirc.org

NOCIRC is "an organization of diverse individuals committed through research, education, and advocacy to securing the birthright of male, female, and intersex infants and children to keep their sex organs intact."

National Vaccine Information Center (NVIC):

http://www.909shot.com

Dedicated to the prevention of vaccine injuries and deaths through public education, NVIC "provides assistance to parents whose children have suffered vaccine reactions; promotes research to evaluate vaccine safety and effectiveness as well as to identify factors which place individuals at high risk for suffering vaccine reactions; and monitors vaccine research, development, policy-making, and legislation. NVIC supports the right of citizens to exercise informed consent and make educated, independent vaccination decisions for themselves and their children."

Weston A. Price Foundation:

http://www.westonaprice.org

The foundation is dedicated to restoring nutrient-dense foods to the human diet through education, research, and activism. It "supports a number of movements that contribute to this objective, including accurate nutrition instruction, organic and biodynamic farming, pasture-feeding of livestock, community-supported farms, honest and informative labeling, prepared par-

enting, and nurturing therapies. Specific goals include establishment of universal access to clean, certified raw milk and a ban on the use of soy formula for infants."

Wholesomebabyfood.com:

http://www.wholesomebabyfood.com

"We hope that babies and parents everywhere might benefit from the great experience of making Fresh, Wholesome, Homemade baby food! For one hour per week, you can make your baby the very best, most nutritious, and most wholesome food that will further provide your baby the very best start!" The website encourages its visitors to *"go forth and puree!"*

Professional Associations and Referral Directories

American Association of Naturopathic Physicians
www.naturopathic.org

American Association of Oriental Medicine
www.aaom.org

American Holistic Medical Association
www.holisticmedicine.org

Council for Homeopathic Certification
www.homeopathicdirectory.com

Holistic Pediatric Association
www.hpakids.org

International Chiropractic Pediatric Association
www.icpa4kids.com

National Center for Homeopathy
www.homeopathic.org

Sources of Homeopathic Medicines and Herbs

Homeopathic Educational Service
www.homeopathic.com, 510-649-0294

Boiron
www.boiron.com, 800-BLUTUBE

Dolisos
www.dolisos.com, 800-DOLISOS

Kan Herbs and Chinese Modular Solutions
www.kanherb.com, 800-543-5233

Crane Herb Company
www.craneherb.com, 800-227-4118

INDEX

A

Abdominal pain. *See also* Stomach
  danger signs, 217
  massage for, 217–218
  symptoms and treatment,
    215–218
Acetaminophen. *See* Fever
  reducers
Acidophilus, 230
Aconitum, 228
Acrylamides, 28
Acupressure, 11. *See also* Massage
Acupuncture, 8, 10, 180, 214
Acyclovir, 221
ADD. *See* Attention Deficit
  Disorder
ADHD. *See* Attention Deficit
  Hyperactivity Disorder
Advertising, 204
Advice, 3, 6–7, 18
Air fresheners, 76–77. *See also*
  Environmental toxins
Alcohol, 62, 73. *See also* Drugs
Alfalfa, 105
Algae, 29, 31, 38, 48, 49, 172
Alimentum, 139–140
All Kinds of Minds Institute, 202
Allergies, 9, 29, 46, 66, 88,
    158–159, 193, 209, 218, 222.
    See also Environmental toxins
  discussed, 177–182

food allergies, 20, 21, 27, 38, 53,
    130, 146, 150, 152, 156,
    170–171, 245–246
  allergenic/toxic foods, 156,
    165–166, 195
Allium cepa, 223
Allopathic medicine. *See also*
  Drugs; Holistic medicine;
  Naturopathic medicine;
  Pediatrician; Vaccine
  compared to holistic medicine,
    4–7, 221
  role of, 7–8
American Academy of Pediatrics,
    35, 52, 87, 116
American Botanical Council, 132
American Dental Association, 84
Amino acids, 153
Anemia. *See also* Iron
  factors affecting, 38, 40, 159–161
  testing for, 7, 152
Anger, 192. *See also* Emotions
Animal products, 42. *See also* Fats;
  Food; Nitrates
  recommendations for, 20, 21, 26,
    29, 31, 153, 160, 161
  eggs, 41, 130–131, 146–147,
    176, 195, 246
Antibiotics, 170, 178–179, 209,
    232–233. *See also* Drugs
  discussed, 80, 158–159
  for strep, 248–249

OTHER NORTH ATLANTIC BOOKS
by Randall Nuestaedter, OMD

Homeopathic Pediatrics: Assessment and Case Management

The Vaccine Guide: Risks and Benefits for Children and Adults

FLU: Alternative Treatments and Prevention